FOOD ALLERGY JOURNAL AND SYMPTOM TRACKER
FOR BREASTFEEDING MOMS AND CHILDREN

Note: A food journal or diary and symptom tracker is a tool to help you and your doctor, it is not a intended to diagnose a food allergy. Always work with your health care professional to identify and treat food allergies.

TO MY SISTER AND MY NIECE.

TRIALED FOODS

FOOD	DATES	PASS	FAIL	NOTES
		☐	☐	
		☐	☐	
		☐	☐	
		☐	☐	
		☐	☐	
		☐	☐	
		☐	☐	
		☐	☐	
		☐	☐	
		☐	☐	
		☐	☐	
		☐	☐	
		☐	☐	
		☐	☐	
		☐	☐	
		☐	☐	
		☐	☐	
		☐	☐	
		☐	☐	
		☐	☐	
		☐	☐	
		☐	☐	
		☐	☐	
		☐	☐	
		☐	☐	
		☐	☐	
		☐	☐	
		☐	☐	
		☐	☐	
		☐	☐	
		☐	☐	
		☐	☐	
		☐	☐	
		☐	☐	
		☐	☐	
		☐	☐	
		☐	☐	
		☐	☐	
		☐	☐	
		☐	☐	
		☐	☐	

TRIALED FOODS

FOOD	DATES	PASS	FAIL	NOTES
		☐	☐	
		☐	☐	
		☐	☐	
		☐	☐	
		☐	☐	
		☐	☐	
		☐	☐	
		☐	☐	
		☐	☐	
		☐	☐	
		☐	☐	
		☐	☐	
		☐	☐	
		☐	☐	
		☐	☐	
		☐	☐	
		☐	☐	
		☐	☐	
		☐	☐	
		☐	☐	
		☐	☐	
		☐	☐	
		☐	☐	
		☐	☐	
		☐	☐	
		☐	☐	
		☐	☐	
		☐	☐	
		☐	☐	
		☐	☐	
		☐	☐	
		☐	☐	
		☐	☐	
		☐	☐	

TRIALED FOODS

FOOD	DATES	PASS	FAIL	NOTES
		☐	☐	
		☐	☐	
		☐	☐	
		☐	☐	
		☐	☐	
		☐	☐	
		☐	☐	
		☐	☐	
		☐	☐	
		☐	☐	
		☐	☐	
		☐	☐	
		☐	☐	
		☐	☐	
		☐	☐	
		☐	☐	
		☐	☐	
		☐	☐	
		☐	☐	
		☐	☐	
		☐	☐	
		☐	☐	
		☐	☐	
		☐	☐	
		☐	☐	
		☐	☐	
		☐	☐	
		☐	☐	
		☐	☐	
		☐	☐	
		☐	☐	
		☐	☐	
		☐	☐	
		☐	☐	
		☐	☐	
		☐	☐	
		☐	☐	
		☐	☐	

SYMPTOMS

		X	NOTES/TIME STARTED	NOTES

SKIN
- ITCHINESS
- HIVES
- RASH
- SWELLING
- REDNESS
- PALENESS
- ECZEMA
- OTHER

THROAT / STOMACH
- DIFFICULTY SWALLOWING
- CHOKING
- REFLUX
- IMMEDIATE VOMITING
- DELAYED VOMITING
- OTHER

NASAL / SINUSES
- STUFFY NOSE
- RUNNY NOSE
- ITCHY THROAT
- HOARSE VOICE
- REPETITIVE COUGHING
- OTHER

LUNGS
- WHEEZING
- SHORTNESS OF BREATH
- DIFFICULTY BREATHING
- OTHER

STOOL
- DIARRHEA
- CONSTIPATION
- BLOODY STOOL
- MUCOUS IN STOOL
- GREEN STOOL
- UNUSUAL ODOR
- OTHER

NEUROLOGICAL
- IRRITABILITY
- HYPERACTIVITY
- INCREASED TANTRUMS
- CLINGINESS
- FAINTING
- DIZZINESS
- EXCESSIVE CRYING
- LETHARGY/FATIGUE
- MOTOR TICS
- SEIZURES
- DIFFICULTY SLEEPING
- FEVER
- LOW TEMPERATURE
- OTHER

DATE _____

MOM'S MEALS

BREAKFAST

SNACK

LUNCH

SNACK

DINNER

SNACK

MEDICATION

CHILD'S MEALS

BREAKFAST

SNACK

LUNCH

SNACK

DINNER

SNACK

MEDICATION

FOOD TRIALING: _____ DAYS TRIALED: _____

SYMPTOMS

		X	NOTES/TIME STARTED	NOTES
SKIN	ITCHINESS			
	HIVES			
	RASH			
	SWELLING			
	REDNESS			
	PALENESS			
	ECZEMA			
	OTHER			
THROAT STOMACH	DIFFICULTY SWALLOWING			
	CHOKING			
	REFLUX			
	IMMEDIATE VOMITING			
	DELAYED VOMITING			
	OTHER			
NASAL SINUSES	STUFFY NOSE			
	RUNNY NOSE			
	ITCHY THROAT			
	HOARSE VOICE			
	REPETITIVE COUGHING			
	OTHER			
LUNGS	WHEEZING			
	SHORTNESS OF BREATH			
	DIFFICULTY BREATHING			
	OTHER			
STOOL	DIARRHEA			
	CONSTIPATION			
	BLOODY STOOL			
	MUCOUS IN STOOL			
	GREEN STOOL			
	UNUSUAL ODOR			
	OTHER			
NEUROLOGICAL	IRRITABILITY			
	HYPERACTIVITY			
	INCREASED TANTRUMS			
	CLINGINESS			
	FAINTING			
	DIZZINESS			
	EXCESSIVE CRYING			
	LETHARGY/FATIGUE			
	MOTOR TICS			
	SEIZURES			
	DIFFICULTY SLEEPING			
	FEVER			
	LOW TEMPERATURE			
	OTHER			

DATE _____

MOM'S MEALS

BREAKFAST

SNACK

LUNCH

SNACK

DINNER

SNACK

MEDICATION

CHILD'S MEALS

BREAKFAST

SNACK

LUNCH

SNACK

DINNER

SNACK

MEDICATION

FOOD TRIALING: _____ DAYS TRIALED: _____

SYMPTOMS

		X	NOTES/TIME STARTED	NOTES
SKIN	ITCHINESS			
	HIVES			
	RASH			
	SWELLING			
	REDNESS			
	PALENESS			
	ECZEMA			
	OTHER			
THROAT STOMACH	DIFFICULTY SWALLOWING			
	CHOKING			
	REFLUX			
	IMMEDIATE VOMITING			
	DELAYED VOMITING			
	OTHER			
NASAL SINUSES	STUFFY NOSE			
	RUNNY NOSE			
	ITCHY THROAT			
	HOARSE VOICE			
	REPETITIVE COUGHING			
	OTHER			
LUNGS	WHEEZING			
	SHORTNESS OF BREATH			
	DIFFICULTY BREATHING			
	OTHER			
STOOL	DIARRHEA			
	CONSTIPATION			
	BLOODY STOOL			
	MUCOUS IN STOOL			
	GREEN STOOL			
	UNUSUAL ODOR			
	OTHER			
NEUROLOGICAL	IRRITABILITY			
	HYPERACTIVITY			
	INCREASED TANTRUMS			
	CLINGINESS			
	FAINTING			
	DIZZINESS			
	EXCESSIVE CRYING			
	LETHARGY/FATIGUE			
	MOTOR TICS			
	SEIZURES			
	DIFFICULTY SLEEPING			
	FEVER			
	LOW TEMPERATURE			
	OTHER			

DATE _____

MOM'S MEALS

BREAKFAST

SNACK
_____
_____
_____

LUNCH

SNACK
_____
_____
_____

DINNER

SNACK
_____
_____

MEDICATION
_____

CHILD'S MEALS

BREAKFAST

SNACK
_____
_____
_____

LUNCH

SNACK
_____
_____
_____

DINNER

SNACK
_____
_____

MEDICATION
_____

FOOD TRIALING: _____ DAYS TRIALED: _____

SYMPTOMS

		X	NOTES/TIME STARTED	NOTES
SKIN	ITCHINESS			
	HIVES			
	RASH			
	SWELLING			
	REDNESS			
	PALENESS			
	ECZEMA			
	OTHER			
THROAT STOMACH	DIFFICULTY SWALLOWING			
	CHOKING			
	REFLUX			
	IMMEDIATE VOMITING			
	DELAYED VOMITING			
	OTHER			
NASAL SINUSES	STUFFY NOSE			
	RUNNY NOSE			
	ITCHY THROAT			
	HOARSE VOICE			
	REPETITIVE COUGHING			
	OTHER			
LUNGS	WHEEZING			
	SHORTNESS OF BREATH			
	DIFFICULTY BREATHING			
	OTHER			
STOOL	DIARRHEA			
	CONSTIPATION			
	BLOODY STOOL			
	MUCOUS IN STOOL			
	GREEN STOOL			
	UNUSUAL ODOR			
	OTHER			
NEUROLOGICAL	IRRITABILITY			
	HYPERACTIVITY			
	INCREASED TANTRUMS			
	CLINGINESS			
	FAINTING			
	DIZZINESS			
	EXCESSIVE CRYING			
	LETHARGY/FATIGUE			
	MOTOR TICS			
	SEIZURES			
	DIFFICULTY SLEEPING			
	FEVER			
	LOW TEMPERATURE			
	OTHER			

DATE _____

MOM'S MEALS

BREAKFAST

SNACK

LUNCH

SNACK

DINNER

SNACK

MEDICATION

CHILD'S MEALS

BREAKFAST

SNACK

LUNCH

SNACK

DINNER

SNACK

MEDICATION

FOOD TRIALING: _____ DAYS TRIALED: _____

SYMPTOMS

		X	NOTES/TIME STARTED	NOTES
SKIN	ITCHINESS			
	HIVES			
	RASH			
	SWELLING			
	REDNESS			
	PALENESS			
	ECZEMA			
	OTHER			
THROAT STOMACH	DIFFICULTY SWALLOWING			
	CHOKING			
	REFLUX			
	IMMEDIATE VOMITING			
	DELAYED VOMITING			
	OTHER			
NASAL SINUSES	STUFFY NOSE			
	RUNNY NOSE			
	ITCHY THROAT			
	HOARSE VOICE			
	REPETITIVE COUGHING			
	OTHER			
LUNGS	WHEEZING			
	SHORTNESS OF BREATH			
	DIFFICULTY BREATHING			
	OTHER			
STOOL	DIARRHEA			
	CONSTIPATION			
	BLOODY STOOL			
	MUCOUS IN STOOL			
	GREEN STOOL			
	UNUSUAL ODOR			
	OTHER			
NEUROLOGICAL	IRRITABILITY			
	HYPERACTIVITY			
	INCREASED TANTRUMS			
	CLINGINESS			
	FAINTING			
	DIZZINESS			
	EXCESSIVE CRYING			
	LETHARGY/FATIGUE			
	MOTOR TICS			
	SEIZURES			
	DIFFICULTY SLEEPING			
	FEVER			
	LOW TEMPERATURE			
	OTHER			

DATE _____

MOM'S MEALS
BREAKFAST

SNACK

LUNCH

SNACK

DINNER

SNACK

MEDICATION

CHILD'S MEALS
BREAKFAST

SNACK

LUNCH

SNACK

DINNER

SNACK

MEDICATION

FOOD TRIALING: _____ DAYS TRIALED: _____

SYMPTOMS

		X	NOTES/TIME STARTED	NOTES

SKIN	ITCHINESS	
	HIVES	
	RASH	
	SWELLING	
	REDNESS	
	PALENESS	
	ECZEMA	
	OTHER	
THROAT STOMACH	DIFFICULTY SWALLOWING	
	CHOKING	
	REFLUX	
	IMMEDIATE VOMITING	
	DELAYED VOMITING	
	OTHER	
NASAL SINUSES	STUFFY NOSE	
	RUNNY NOSE	
	ITCHY THROAT	
	HOARSE VOICE	
	REPETITIVE COUGHING	
	OTHER	
LUNGS	WHEEZING	
	SHORTNESS OF BREATH	
	DIFFICULTY BREATHING	
	OTHER	
STOOL	DIARRHEA	
	CONSTIPATION	
	BLOODY STOOL	
	MUCOUS IN STOOL	
	GREEN STOOL	
	UNUSUAL ODOR	
	OTHER	
NEUROLOGICAL	IRRITABILITY	
	HYPERACTIVITY	
	INCREASED TANTRUMS	
	CLINGINESS	
	FAINTING	
	DIZZINESS	
	EXCESSIVE CRYING	
	LETHARGY/FATIGUE	
	MOTOR TICS	
	SEIZURES	
	DIFFICULTY SLEEPING	
	FEVER	
	LOW TEMPERATURE	
	OTHER	

DATE _____

MOM'S MEALS

BREAKFAST

SNACK

LUNCH

SNACK

DINNER

SNACK

MEDICATION

CHILD'S MEALS

BREAKFAST

SNACK

LUNCH

SNACK

DINNER

SNACK

MEDICATION

FOOD TRIALING: _____ DAYS TRIALED: _____

SYMPTOMS

		X	NOTES/TIME STARTED	NOTES
SKIN	ITCHINESS			
	HIVES			
	RASH			
	SWELLING			
	REDNESS			
	PALENESS			
	ECZEMA			
	OTHER			
THROAT / STOMACH	DIFFICULTY SWALLOWING			
	CHOKING			
	REFLUX			
	IMMEDIATE VOMITING			
	DELAYED VOMITING			
	OTHER			
NASAL SINUSES	STUFFY NOSE			
	RUNNY NOSE			
	ITCHY THROAT			
	HOARSE VOICE			
	REPETITIVE COUGHING			
	OTHER			
LUNGS	WHEEZING			
	SHORTNESS OF BREATH			
	DIFFICULTY BREATHING			
	OTHER			
STOOL	DIARRHEA			
	CONSTIPATION			
	BLOODY STOOL			
	MUCOUS IN STOOL			
	GREEN STOOL			
	UNUSUAL ODOR			
	OTHER			
NEUROLOGICAL	IRRITABILITY			
	HYPERACTIVITY			
	INCREASED TANTRUMS			
	CLINGINESS			
	FAINTING			
	DIZZINESS			
	EXCESSIVE CRYING			
	LETHARGY/FATIGUE			
	MOTOR TICS			
	SEIZURES			
	DIFFICULTY SLEEPING			
	FEVER			
	LOW TEMPERATURE			
	OTHER			

DATE _____

MOM'S MEALS
BREAKFAST

SNACK

LUNCH

SNACK

DINNER

SNACK

MEDICATION

CHILD'S MEALS
BREAKFAST

SNACK

LUNCH

SNACK

DINNER

SNACK

MEDICATION

FOOD TRIALING: _____ DAYS TRIALED: _____

SYMPTOMS

		X	NOTES/TIME STARTED	NOTES
SKIN	ITCHINESS			
	HIVES			
	RASH			
	SWELLING			
	REDNESS			
	PALENESS			
	ECZEMA			
	OTHER			
THROAT STOMACH	DIFFICULTY SWALLOWING			
	CHOKING			
	REFLUX			
	IMMEDIATE VOMITING			
	DELAYED VOMITING			
	OTHER			
NASAL SINUSES	STUFFY NOSE			
	RUNNY NOSE			
	ITCHY THROAT			
	HOARSE VOICE			
	REPETITIVE COUGHING			
	OTHER			
LUNGS	WHEEZING			
	SHORTNESS OF BREATH			
	DIFFICULTY BREATHING			
	OTHER			
STOOL	DIARRHEA			
	CONSTIPATION			
	BLOODY STOOL			
	MUCOUS IN STOOL			
	GREEN STOOL			
	UNUSUAL ODOR			
	OTHER			
NEUROLOGICAL	IRRITABILITY			
	HYPERACTIVITY			
	INCREASED TANTRUMS			
	CLINGINESS			
	FAINTING			
	DIZZINESS			
	EXCESSIVE CRYING			
	LETHARGY/FATIGUE			
	MOTOR TICS			
	SEIZURES			
	DIFFICULTY SLEEPING			
	FEVER			
	LOW TEMPERATURE			
	OTHER			

DATE _____

MOM'S MEALS

BREAKFAST

SNACK

LUNCH

SNACK

DINNER

SNACK

MEDICATION

CHILD'S MEALS

BREAKFAST

SNACK

LUNCH

SNACK

DINNER

SNACK

MEDICATION

FOOD TRIALING: _____ DAYS TRIALED: _____

SYMPTOMS

		X	NOTES/TIME STARTED	NOTES
SKIN	ITCHINESS			
	HIVES			
	RASH			
	SWELLING			
	REDNESS			
	PALENESS			
	ECZEMA			
	OTHER			
THROAT STOMACH	DIFFICULTY SWALLOWING			
	CHOKING			
	REFLUX			
	IMMEDIATE VOMITING			
	DELAYED VOMITING			
	OTHER			
NASAL SINUSES	STUFFY NOSE			
	RUNNY NOSE			
	ITCHY THROAT			
	HOARSE VOICE			
	REPETITIVE COUGHING			
	OTHER			
LUNGS	WHEEZING			
	SHORTNESS OF BREATH			
	DIFFICULTY BREATHING			
	OTHER			
STOOL	DIARRHEA			
	CONSTIPATION			
	BLOODY STOOL			
	MUCOUS IN STOOL			
	GREEN STOOL			
	UNUSUAL ODOR			
	OTHER			
NEUROLOGICAL	IRRITABILITY			
	HYPERACTIVITY			
	INCREASED TANTRUMS			
	CLINGINESS			
	FAINTING			
	DIZZINESS			
	EXCESSIVE CRYING			
	LETHARGY/FATIGUE			
	MOTOR TICS			
	SEIZURES			
	DIFFICULTY SLEEPING			
	FEVER			
	LOW TEMPERATURE			
	OTHER			

DATE _____

MOM'S MEALS

BREAKFAST

SNACK

LUNCH

SNACK

DINNER

SNACK

MEDICATION

CHILD'S MEALS

BREAKFAST

SNACK

LUNCH

SNACK

DINNER

SNACK

MEDICATION

FOOD TRIALING: _____   DAYS TRIALED: _____

SYMPTOMS

	Symptom	X NOTES/TIME STARTED	NOTES
SKIN	ITCHINESS		
	HIVES		
	RASH		
	SWELLING		
	REDNESS		
	PALENESS		
	ECZEMA		
	OTHER		
THROAT STOMACH	DIFFICULTY SWALLOWING		
	CHOKING		
	REFLUX		
	IMMEDIATE VOMITING		
	DELAYED VOMITING		
	OTHER		
NASAL SINUSES	STUFFY NOSE		
	RUNNY NOSE		
	ITCHY THROAT		
	HOARSE VOICE		
	REPETITIVE COUGHING		
	OTHER		
LUNGS	WHEEZING		
	SHORTNESS OF BREATH		
	DIFFICULTY BREATHING		
	OTHER		
STOOL	DIARRHEA		
	CONSTIPATION		
	BLOODY STOOL		
	MUCOUS IN STOOL		
	GREEN STOOL		
	UNUSUAL ODOR		
	OTHER		
NEUROLOGICAL	IRRITABILITY		
	HYPERACTIVITY		
	INCREASED TANTRUMS		
	CLINGINESS		
	FAINTING		
	DIZZINESS		
	EXCESSIVE CRYING		
	LETHARGY/FATIGUE		
	MOTOR TICS		
	SEIZURES		
	DIFFICULTY SLEEPING		
	FEVER		
	LOW TEMPERATURE		
	OTHER		

DATE _____

MOM'S MEALS

BREAKFAST

SNACK

LUNCH

SNACK

DINNER

SNACK

MEDICATION

CHILD'S MEALS

BREAKFAST

SNACK

LUNCH

SNACK

DINNER

SNACK

MEDICATION

FOOD TRIALING: _____   DAYS TRIALED: _____

SYMPTOMS

		X	NOTES/TIME STARTED	NOTES
SKIN	ITCHINESS			
	HIVES			
	RASH			
	SWELLING			
	REDNESS			
	PALENESS			
	ECZEMA			
	OTHER			
THROAT STOMACH	DIFFICULTY SWALLOWING			
	CHOKING			
	REFLUX			
	IMMEDIATE VOMITING			
	DELAYED VOMITING			
	OTHER			
NASAL SINUSES	STUFFY NOSE			
	RUNNY NOSE			
	ITCHY THROAT			
	HOARSE VOICE			
	REPETITIVE COUGHING			
	OTHER			
LUNGS	WHEEZING			
	SHORTNESS OF BREATH			
	DIFFICULTY BREATHING			
	OTHER			
STOOL	DIARRHEA			
	CONSTIPATION			
	BLOODY STOOL			
	MUCOUS IN STOOL			
	GREEN STOOL			
	UNUSUAL ODOR			
	OTHER			
NEUROLOGICAL	IRRITABILITY			
	HYPERACTIVITY			
	INCREASED TANTRUMS			
	CLINGINESS			
	FAINTING			
	DIZZINESS			
	EXCESSIVE CRYING			
	LETHARGY/FATIGUE			
	MOTOR TICS			
	SEIZURES			
	DIFFICULTY SLEEPING			
	FEVER			
	LOW TEMPERATURE			
	OTHER			

DATE _____

MOM'S MEALS

BREAKFAST

SNACK

LUNCH

SNACK

DINNER

SNACK

MEDICATION

CHILD'S MEALS

BREAKFAST

SNACK

LUNCH

SNACK

DINNER

SNACK

MEDICATION

FOOD TRIALING: _____ DAYS TRIALED: _____

SYMPTOMS

		X	NOTES/TIME STARTED	NOTES
SKIN	ITCHINESS			
	HIVES			
	RASH			
	SWELLING			
	REDNESS			
	PALENESS			
	ECZEMA			
	OTHER			
THROAT STOMACH	DIFFICULTY SWALLOWING			
	CHOKING			
	REFLUX			
	IMMEDIATE VOMITING			
	DELAYED VOMITING			
	OTHER			
NASAL SINUSES	STUFFY NOSE			
	RUNNY NOSE			
	ITCHY THROAT			
	HOARSE VOICE			
	REPETITIVE COUGHING			
	OTHER			
LUNGS	WHEEZING			
	SHORTNESS OF BREATH			
	DIFFICULTY BREATHING			
	OTHER			
STOOL	DIARRHEA			
	CONSTIPATION			
	BLOODY STOOL			
	MUCOUS IN STOOL			
	GREEN STOOL			
	UNUSUAL ODOR			
	OTHER			
NEUROLOGICAL	IRRITABILITY			
	HYPERACTIVITY			
	INCREASED TANTRUMS			
	CLINGINESS			
	FAINTING			
	DIZZINESS			
	EXCESSIVE CRYING			
	LETHARGY/FATIGUE			
	MOTOR TICS			
	SEIZURES			
	DIFFICULTY SLEEPING			
	FEVER			
	LOW TEMPERATURE			
	OTHER			

DATE _____

MOM'S MEALS

BREAKFAST

SNACK

LUNCH

SNACK

DINNER

SNACK

MEDICATION

CHILD'S MEALS

BREAKFAST

SNACK

LUNCH

SNACK

DINNER

SNACK

MEDICATION

FOOD TRIALING: _____ DAYS TRIALED: _____

SYMPTOMS

		X	NOTES/TIME STARTED	NOTES
SKIN	ITCHINESS			
	HIVES			
	RASH			
	SWELLING			
	REDNESS			
	PALENESS			
	ECZEMA			
	OTHER			
THROAT STOMACH	DIFFICULTY SWALLOWING			
	CHOKING			
	REFLUX			
	IMMEDIATE VOMITING			
	DELAYED VOMITING			
	OTHER			
NASAL SINUSES	STUFFY NOSE			
	RUNNY NOSE			
	ITCHY THROAT			
	HOARSE VOICE			
	REPETITIVE COUGHING			
	OTHER			
LUNGS	WHEEZING			
	SHORTNESS OF BREATH			
	DIFFICULTY BREATHING			
	OTHER			
STOOL	DIARRHEA			
	CONSTIPATION			
	BLOODY STOOL			
	MUCOUS IN STOOL			
	GREEN STOOL			
	UNUSUAL ODOR			
	OTHER			
NEUROLOGICAL	IRRITABILITY			
	HYPERACTIVITY			
	INCREASED TANTRUMS			
	CLINGINESS			
	FAINTING			
	DIZZINESS			
	EXCESSIVE CRYING			
	LETHARGY/FATIGUE			
	MOTOR TICS			
	SEIZURES			
	DIFFICULTY SLEEPING			
	FEVER			
	LOW TEMPERATURE			
	OTHER			

DATE _____

MOM'S MEALS

BREAKFAST

SNACK

LUNCH

SNACK

DINNER

SNACK

MEDICATION

CHILD'S MEALS

BREAKFAST

SNACK

LUNCH

SNACK

DINNER

SNACK

MEDICATION

FOOD TRIALING: _____ DAYS TRIALED: _____

SYMPTOMS

		X	NOTES/TIME STARTED	NOTES
SKIN	ITCHINESS			
	HIVES			
	RASH			
	SWELLING			
	REDNESS			
	PALENESS			
	ECZEMA			
	OTHER			
THROAT STOMACH	DIFFICULTY SWALLOWING			
	CHOKING			
	REFLUX			
	IMMEDIATE VOMITING			
	DELAYED VOMITING			
	OTHER			
NASAL SINUSES	STUFFY NOSE			
	RUNNY NOSE			
	ITCHY THROAT			
	HOARSE VOICE			
	REPETITIVE COUGHING			
	OTHER			
LUNGS	WHEEZING			
	SHORTNESS OF BREATH			
	DIFFICULTY BREATHING			
	OTHER			
STOOL	DIARRHEA			
	CONSTIPATION			
	BLOODY STOOL			
	MUCOUS IN STOOL			
	GREEN STOOL			
	UNUSUAL ODOR			
	OTHER			
NEUROLOGICAL	IRRITABILITY			
	HYPERACTIVITY			
	INCREASED TANTRUMS			
	CLINGINESS			
	FAINTING			
	DIZZINESS			
	EXCESSIVE CRYING			
	LETHARGY/FATIGUE			
	MOTOR TICS			
	SEIZURES			
	DIFFICULTY SLEEPING			
	FEVER			
	LOW TEMPERATURE			
	OTHER			

DATE _____

MOM'S MEALS
BREAKFAST

SNACK
_____
_____
_____

LUNCH

SNACK
_____
_____
_____

DINNER

SNACK
_____

MEDICATION
_____

CHILD'S MEALS
BREAKFAST

SNACK
_____
_____
_____

LUNCH

SNACK
_____
_____
_____

DINNER

SNACK
_____

MEDICATION
_____

FOOD TRIALING: _____ DAYS TRIALED: _____

SYMPTOMS

		X	NOTES/TIME STARTED	NOTES

	Symptom	X	NOTES/TIME STARTED	NOTES
SKIN	ITCHINESS			
	HIVES			
	RASH			
	SWELLING			
	REDNESS			
	PALENESS			
	ECZEMA			
	OTHER			
THROAT STOMACH	DIFFICULTY SWALLOWING			
	CHOKING			
	REFLUX			
	IMMEDIATE VOMITING			
	DELAYED VOMITING			
	OTHER			
NASAL SINUSES	STUFFY NOSE			
	RUNNY NOSE			
	ITCHY THROAT			
	HOARSE VOICE			
	REPETITIVE COUGHING			
	OTHER			
LUNGS	WHEEZING			
	SHORTNESS OF BREATH			
	DIFFICULTY BREATHING			
	OTHER			
STOOL	DIARRHEA			
	CONSTIPATION			
	BLOODY STOOL			
	MUCOUS IN STOOL			
	GREEN STOOL			
	UNUSUAL ODOR			
	OTHER			
NEUROLOGICAL	IRRITABILITY			
	HYPERACTIVITY			
	INCREASED TANTRUMS			
	CLINGINESS			
	FAINTING			
	DIZZINESS			
	EXCESSIVE CRYING			
	LETHARGY/FATIGUE			
	MOTOR TICS			
	SEIZURES			
	DIFFICULTY SLEEPING			
	FEVER			
	LOW TEMPERATURE			
	OTHER			

DATE _____

MOM'S MEALS
BREAKFAST

SNACK

LUNCH

SNACK

DINNER

SNACK

MEDICATION

CHILD'S MEALS
BREAKFAST

SNACK

LUNCH

SNACK

DINNER

SNACK

MEDICATION

FOOD TRIALING: _____ DAYS TRIALED: _____

SYMPTOMS

		X	NOTES/TIME STARTED	NOTES
SKIN	ITCHINESS			
	HIVES			
	RASH			
	SWELLING			
	REDNESS			
	PALENESS			
	ECZEMA			
	OTHER			
THROAT STOMACH	DIFFICULTY SWALLOWING			
	CHOKING			
	REFLUX			
	IMMEDIATE VOMITING			
	DELAYED VOMITING			
	OTHER			
NASAL SINUSES	STUFFY NOSE			
	RUNNY NOSE			
	ITCHY THROAT			
	HOARSE VOICE			
	REPETITIVE COUGHING			
	OTHER			
LUNGS	WHEEZING			
	SHORTNESS OF BREATH			
	DIFFICULTY BREATHING			
	OTHER			
STOOL	DIARRHEA			
	CONSTIPATION			
	BLOODY STOOL			
	MUCOUS IN STOOL			
	GREEN STOOL			
	UNUSUAL ODOR			
	OTHER			
NEUROLOGICAL	IRRITABILITY			
	HYPERACTIVITY			
	INCREASED TANTRUMS			
	CLINGINESS			
	FAINTING			
	DIZZINESS			
	EXCESSIVE CRYING			
	LETHARGY/FATIGUE			
	MOTOR TICS			
	SEIZURES			
	DIFFICULTY SLEEPING			
	FEVER			
	LOW TEMPERATURE			
	OTHER			

DATE _____

MOM'S MEALS

BREAKFAST

SNACK
_____

LUNCH

SNACK
_____

DINNER

SNACK
_____

MEDICATION

CHILD'S MEALS

BREAKFAST

SNACK
_____

LUNCH

SNACK
_____

DINNER

SNACK
_____

MEDICATION

FOOD TRIALING: _____ DAYS TRIALED: _____

SYMPTOMS

		X	NOTES/TIME STARTED	NOTES

	Symptom	X	NOTES/TIME STARTED	NOTES
SKIN	ITCHINESS			
	HIVES			
	RASH			
	SWELLING			
	REDNESS			
	PALENESS			
	ECZEMA			
	OTHER			
THROAT STOMACH	DIFFICULTY SWALLOWING			
	CHOKING			
	REFLUX			
	IMMEDIATE VOMITING			
	DELAYED VOMITING			
	OTHER			
NASAL SINUSES	STUFFY NOSE			
	RUNNY NOSE			
	ITCHY THROAT			
	HOARSE VOICE			
	REPETITIVE COUGHING			
	OTHER			
LUNGS	WHEEZING			
	SHORTNESS OF BREATH			
	DIFFICULTY BREATHING			
	OTHER			
STOOL	DIARRHEA			
	CONSTIPATION			
	BLOODY STOOL			
	MUCOUS IN STOOL			
	GREEN STOOL			
	UNUSUAL ODOR			
	OTHER			
NEUROLOGICAL	IRRITABILITY			
	HYPERACTIVITY			
	INCREASED TANTRUMS			
	CLINGINESS			
	FAINTING			
	DIZZINESS			
	EXCESSIVE CRYING			
	LETHARGY/FATIGUE			
	MOTOR TICS			
	SEIZURES			
	DIFFICULTY SLEEPING			
	FEVER			
	LOW TEMPERATURE			
	OTHER			

DATE _____

MOM'S MEALS

BREAKFAST

SNACK

LUNCH

SNACK

DINNER

SNACK

MEDICATION

CHILD'S MEALS

BREAKFAST

SNACK

LUNCH

SNACK

DINNER

SNACK

MEDICATION

FOOD TRIALING: _____   DAYS TRIALED: _____

SYMPTOMS

	X	NOTES/TIME STARTED	NOTES

SKIN	ITCHINESS			
	HIVES			
	RASH			
	SWELLING			
	REDNESS			
	PALENESS			
	ECZEMA			
	OTHER			
THROAT STOMACH	DIFFICULTY SWALLOWING			
	CHOKING			
	REFLUX			
	IMMEDIATE VOMITING			
	DELAYED VOMITING			
	OTHER			
NASAL SINUSES	STUFFY NOSE			
	RUNNY NOSE			
	ITCHY THROAT			
	HOARSE VOICE			
	REPETITIVE COUGHING			
	OTHER			
LUNGS	WHEEZING			
	SHORTNESS OF BREATH			
	DIFFICULTY BREATHING			
	OTHER			
STOOL	DIARRHEA			
	CONSTIPATION			
	BLOODY STOOL			
	MUCOUS IN STOOL			
	GREEN STOOL			
	UNUSUAL ODOR			
	OTHER			
NEUROLOGICAL	IRRITABILITY			
	HYPERACTIVITY			
	INCREASED TANTRUMS			
	CLINGINESS			
	FAINTING			
	DIZZINESS			
	EXCESSIVE CRYING			
	LETHARGY/FATIGUE			
	MOTOR TICS			
	SEIZURES			
	DIFFICULTY SLEEPING			
	FEVER			
	LOW TEMPERATURE			
	OTHER			

DATE _____

MOM'S MEALS

BREAKFAST

SNACK

LUNCH

SNACK

DINNER

SNACK

MEDICATION

CHILD'S MEALS

BREAKFAST

SNACK

LUNCH

SNACK

DINNER

SNACK

MEDICATION

FOOD TRIALING: _____ DAYS TRIALED: _____

SYMPTOMS

		X	NOTES/TIME STARTED	NOTES

SKIN	ITCHINESS		
	HIVES		
	RASH		
	SWELLING		
	REDNESS		
	PALENESS		
	ECZEMA		
	OTHER		
THROAT STOMACH	DIFFICULTY SWALLOWING		
	CHOKING		
	REFLUX		
	IMMEDIATE VOMITING		
	DELAYED VOMITING		
	OTHER		
NASAL SINUSES	STUFFY NOSE		
	RUNNY NOSE		
	ITCHY THROAT		
	HOARSE VOICE		
	REPETITIVE COUGHING		
	OTHER		
LUNGS	WHEEZING		
	SHORTNESS OF BREATH		
	DIFFICULTY BREATHING		
	OTHER		
STOOL	DIARRHEA		
	CONSTIPATION		
	BLOODY STOOL		
	MUCOUS IN STOOL		
	GREEN STOOL		
	UNUSUAL ODOR		
	OTHER		
NEUROLOGICAL	IRRITABILITY		
	HYPERACTIVITY		
	INCREASED TANTRUMS		
	CLINGINESS		
	FAINTING		
	DIZZINESS		
	EXCESSIVE CRYING		
	LETHARGY/FATIGUE		
	MOTOR TICS		
	SEIZURES		
	DIFFICULTY SLEEPING		
	FEVER		
	LOW TEMPERATURE		
	OTHER		

DATE _____

MOM'S MEALS
BREAKFAST

SNACK

LUNCH

SNACK

DINNER

SNACK

MEDICATION

CHILD'S MEALS
BREAKFAST

SNACK

LUNCH

SNACK

DINNER

SNACK

MEDICATION

FOOD TRIALING: _____   DAYS TRIALED: _____

SYMPTOMS

		X	NOTES/TIME STARTED	NOTES
SKIN	ITCHINESS			
	HIVES			
	RASH			
	SWELLING			
	REDNESS			
	PALENESS			
	ECZEMA			
	OTHER			
THROAT STOMACH	DIFFICULTY SWALLOWING			
	CHOKING			
	REFLUX			
	IMMEDIATE VOMITING			
	DELAYED VOMITING			
	OTHER			
NASAL SINUSES	STUFFY NOSE			
	RUNNY NOSE			
	ITCHY THROAT			
	HOARSE VOICE			
	REPETITIVE COUGHING			
	OTHER			
LUNGS	WHEEZING			
	SHORTNESS OF BREATH			
	DIFFICULTY BREATHING			
	OTHER			
STOOL	DIARRHEA			
	CONSTIPATION			
	BLOODY STOOL			
	MUCOUS IN STOOL			
	GREEN STOOL			
	UNUSUAL ODOR			
	OTHER			
NEUROLOGICAL	IRRITABILITY			
	HYPERACTIVITY			
	INCREASED TANTRUMS			
	CLINGINESS			
	FAINTING			
	DIZZINESS			
	EXCESSIVE CRYING			
	LETHARGY/FATIGUE			
	MOTOR TICS			
	SEIZURES			
	DIFFICULTY SLEEPING			
	FEVER			
	LOW TEMPERATURE			
	OTHER			

DATE _____

MOM'S MEALS

BREAKFAST

SNACK

LUNCH

SNACK

DINNER

SNACK

MEDICATION

CHILD'S MEALS

BREAKFAST

SNACK

LUNCH

SNACK

DINNER

SNACK

MEDICATION

FOOD TRIALING: _____ DAYS TRIALED: _____

SYMPTOMS

		X	NOTES/TIME STARTED	NOTES
SKIN	ITCHINESS			
	HIVES			
	RASH			
	SWELLING			
	REDNESS			
	PALENESS			
	ECZEMA			
	OTHER			
THROAT STOMACH	DIFFICULTY SWALLOWING			
	CHOKING			
	REFLUX			
	IMMEDIATE VOMITING			
	DELAYED VOMITING			
	OTHER			
NASAL SINUSES	STUFFY NOSE			
	RUNNY NOSE			
	ITCHY THROAT			
	HOARSE VOICE			
	REPETITIVE COUGHING			
	OTHER			
LUNGS	WHEEZING			
	SHORTNESS OF BREATH			
	DIFFICULTY BREATHING			
	OTHER			
STOOL	DIARRHEA			
	CONSTIPATION			
	BLOODY STOOL			
	MUCOUS IN STOOL			
	GREEN STOOL			
	UNUSUAL ODOR			
	OTHER			
NEUROLOGICAL	IRRITABILITY			
	HYPERACTIVITY			
	INCREASED TANTRUMS			
	CLINGINESS			
	FAINTING			
	DIZZINESS			
	EXCESSIVE CRYING			
	LETHARGY/FATIGUE			
	MOTOR TICS			
	SEIZURES			
	DIFFICULTY SLEEPING			
	FEVER			
	LOW TEMPERATURE			
	OTHER			

DATE _____

MOM'S MEALS

BREAKFAST

SNACK

LUNCH

SNACK

DINNER

SNACK

MEDICATION

CHILD'S MEALS

BREAKFAST

SNACK

LUNCH

SNACK

DINNER

SNACK

MEDICATION

FOOD TRIALING: _____   DAYS TRIALED: _____

SYMPTOMS

	Symptoms	X	NOTES/TIME STARTED	NOTES
SKIN	ITCHINESS			
	HIVES			
	RASH			
	SWELLING			
	REDNESS			
	PALENESS			
	ECZEMA			
	OTHER			
THROAT STOMACH	DIFFICULTY SWALLOWING			
	CHOKING			
	REFLUX			
	IMMEDIATE VOMITING			
	DELAYED VOMITING			
	OTHER			
NASAL SINUSES	STUFFY NOSE			
	RUNNY NOSE			
	ITCHY THROAT			
	HOARSE VOICE			
	REPETITIVE COUGHING			
	OTHER			
LUNGS	WHEEZING			
	SHORTNESS OF BREATH			
	DIFFICULTY BREATHING			
	OTHER			
STOOL	DIARRHEA			
	CONSTIPATION			
	BLOODY STOOL			
	MUCOUS IN STOOL			
	GREEN STOOL			
	UNUSUAL ODOR			
	OTHER			
NEUROLOGICAL	IRRITABILITY			
	HYPERACTIVITY			
	INCREASED TANTRUMS			
	CLINGINESS			
	FAINTING			
	DIZZINESS			
	EXCESSIVE CRYING			
	LETHARGY/FATIGUE			
	MOTOR TICS			
	SEIZURES			
	DIFFICULTY SLEEPING			
	FEVER			
	LOW TEMPERATURE			
	OTHER			

DATE _____

MOM'S MEALS

BREAKFAST

SNACK

LUNCH

SNACK

DINNER

SNACK

MEDICATION

CHILD'S MEALS

BREAKFAST

SNACK

LUNCH

SNACK

DINNER

SNACK

MEDICATION

FOOD TRIALING: _____ DAYS TRIALED: _____

SYMPTOMS

		X	NOTES/TIME STARTED	NOTES
SKIN	ITCHINESS			
	HIVES			
	RASH			
	SWELLING			
	REDNESS			
	PALENESS			
	ECZEMA			
	OTHER			
THROAT STOMACH	DIFFICULTY SWALLOWING			
	CHOKING			
	REFLUX			
	IMMEDIATE VOMITING			
	DELAYED VOMITING			
	OTHER			
NASAL SINUSES	STUFFY NOSE			
	RUNNY NOSE			
	ITCHY THROAT			
	HOARSE VOICE			
	REPETITIVE COUGHING			
	OTHER			
LUNGS	WHEEZING			
	SHORTNESS OF BREATH			
	DIFFICULTY BREATHING			
	OTHER			
STOOL	DIARRHEA			
	CONSTIPATION			
	BLOODY STOOL			
	MUCOUS IN STOOL			
	GREEN STOOL			
	UNUSUAL ODOR			
	OTHER			
NEUROLOGICAL	IRRITABILITY			
	HYPERACTIVITY			
	INCREASED TANTRUMS			
	CLINGINESS			
	FAINTING			
	DIZZINESS			
	EXCESSIVE CRYING			
	LETHARGY/FATIGUE			
	MOTOR TICS			
	SEIZURES			
	DIFFICULTY SLEEPING			
	FEVER			
	LOW TEMPERATURE			
	OTHER			

DATE _____

MOM'S MEALS
BREAKFAST

SNACK

LUNCH

SNACK

DINNER

SNACK

MEDICATION

CHILD'S MEALS
BREAKFAST

SNACK

LUNCH

SNACK

DINNER

SNACK

MEDICATION

FOOD TRIALING: _____ DAYS TRIALED: _____

SYMPTOMS

		X	NOTES/TIME STARTED	NOTES

SKIN
ITCHINESS		
HIVES		
RASH		
SWELLING		
REDNESS		
PALENESS		
ECZEMA		
OTHER		

THROAT / STOMACH
DIFFICULTY SWALLOWING		
CHOKING		
REFLUX		
IMMEDIATE VOMITING		
DELAYED VOMITING		
OTHER		

NASAL / SINUSES
STUFFY NOSE		
RUNNY NOSE		
ITCHY THROAT		
HOARSE VOICE		
REPETITIVE COUGHING		
OTHER		

LUNGS
WHEEZING		
SHORTNESS OF BREATH		
DIFFICULTY BREATHING		
OTHER		

STOOL
DIARRHEA		
CONSTIPATION		
BLOODY STOOL		
MUCOUS IN STOOL		
GREEN STOOL		
UNUSUAL ODOR		
OTHER		

NEUROLOGICAL
IRRITABILITY		
HYPERACTIVITY		
INCREASED TANTRUMS		
CLINGINESS		
FAINTING		
DIZZINESS		
EXCESSIVE CRYING		
LETHARGY/FATIGUE		
MOTOR TICS		
SEIZURES		
DIFFICULTY SLEEPING		
FEVER		
LOW TEMPERATURE		
OTHER		

DATE _____

MOM'S MEALS

BREAKFAST

SNACK

LUNCH

SNACK

DINNER

SNACK

MEDICATION

CHILD'S MEALS

BREAKFAST

SNACK

LUNCH

SNACK

DINNER

SNACK

MEDICATION

FOOD TRIALING: _____ DAYS TRIALED: _____

SYMPTOMS

		X	NOTES/TIME STARTED	NOTES
SKIN	ITCHINESS			
	HIVES			
	RASH			
	SWELLING			
	REDNESS			
	PALENESS			
	ECZEMA			
	OTHER			
THROAT STOMACH	DIFFICULTY SWALLOWING			
	CHOKING			
	REFLUX			
	IMMEDIATE VOMITING			
	DELAYED VOMITING			
	OTHER			
NASAL SINUSES	STUFFY NOSE			
	RUNNY NOSE			
	ITCHY THROAT			
	HOARSE VOICE			
	REPETITIVE COUGHING			
	OTHER			
LUNGS	WHEEZING			
	SHORTNESS OF BREATH			
	DIFFICULTY BREATHING			
	OTHER			
STOOL	DIARRHEA			
	CONSTIPATION			
	BLOODY STOOL			
	MUCOUS IN STOOL			
	GREEN STOOL			
	UNUSUAL ODOR			
	OTHER			
NEUROLOGICAL	IRRITABILITY			
	HYPERACTIVITY			
	INCREASED TANTRUMS			
	CLINGINESS			
	FAINTING			
	DIZZINESS			
	EXCESSIVE CRYING			
	LETHARGY/FATIGUE			
	MOTOR TICS			
	SEIZURES			
	DIFFICULTY SLEEPING			
	FEVER			
	LOW TEMPERATURE			
	OTHER			

DATE _____

MOM'S MEALS

BREAKFAST

SNACK

LUNCH

SNACK

DINNER

SNACK

MEDICATION

CHILD'S MEALS

BREAKFAST

SNACK

LUNCH

SNACK

DINNER

SNACK

MEDICATION

FOOD TRIALING: _____ DAYS TRIALED: _____

SYMPTOMS

		X	NOTES/TIME STARTED	NOTES
SKIN	ITCHINESS			
	HIVES			
	RASH			
	SWELLING			
	REDNESS			
	PALENESS			
	ECZEMA			
	OTHER			
THROAT STOMACH	DIFFICULTY SWALLOWING			
	CHOKING			
	REFLUX			
	IMMEDIATE VOMITING			
	DELAYED VOMITING			
	OTHER			
NASAL SINUSES	STUFFY NOSE			
	RUNNY NOSE			
	ITCHY THROAT			
	HOARSE VOICE			
	REPETITIVE COUGHING			
	OTHER			
LUNGS	WHEEZING			
	SHORTNESS OF BREATH			
	DIFFICULTY BREATHING			
	OTHER			
STOOL	DIARRHEA			
	CONSTIPATION			
	BLOODY STOOL			
	MUCOUS IN STOOL			
	GREEN STOOL			
	UNUSUAL ODOR			
	OTHER			
NEUROLOGICAL	IRRITABILITY			
	HYPERACTIVITY			
	INCREASED TANTRUMS			
	CLINGINESS			
	FAINTING			
	DIZZINESS			
	EXCESSIVE CRYING			
	LETHARGY/FATIGUE			
	MOTOR TICS			
	SEIZURES			
	DIFFICULTY SLEEPING			
	FEVER			
	LOW TEMPERATURE			
	OTHER			

DATE _____

MOM'S MEALS
BREAKFAST

CHILD'S MEALS
BREAKFAST

SNACK _____

SNACK _____

LUNCH

LUNCH

SNACK _____

SNACK _____

DINNER

DINNER

SNACK _____

SNACK _____

MEDICATION

MEDICATION

FOOD TRIALING: _____ DAYS TRIALED: _____

SYMPTOMS

		X	NOTES/TIME STARTED	NOTES
SKIN	ITCHINESS			
	HIVES			
	RASH			
	SWELLING			
	REDNESS			
	PALENESS			
	ECZEMA			
	OTHER			
THROAT STOMACH	DIFFICULTY SWALLOWING			
	CHOKING			
	REFLUX			
	IMMEDIATE VOMITING			
	DELAYED VOMITING			
	OTHER			
NASAL SINUSES	STUFFY NOSE			
	RUNNY NOSE			
	ITCHY THROAT			
	HOARSE VOICE			
	REPETITIVE COUGHING			
	OTHER			
LUNGS	WHEEZING			
	SHORTNESS OF BREATH			
	DIFFICULTY BREATHING			
	OTHER			
STOOL	DIARRHEA			
	CONSTIPATION			
	BLOODY STOOL			
	MUCOUS IN STOOL			
	GREEN STOOL			
	UNUSUAL ODOR			
	OTHER			
NEUROLOGICAL	IRRITABILITY			
	HYPERACTIVITY			
	INCREASED TANTRUMS			
	CLINGINESS			
	FAINTING			
	DIZZINESS			
	EXCESSIVE CRYING			
	LETHARGY/FATIGUE			
	MOTOR TICS			
	SEIZURES			
	DIFFICULTY SLEEPING			
	FEVER			
	LOW TEMPERATURE			
	OTHER			

DATE _____

MOM'S MEALS
BREAKFAST

SNACK
_____
_____

LUNCH

SNACK
_____
_____

DINNER

SNACK
_____
_____

MEDICATION

CHILD'S MEALS
BREAKFAST

SNACK
_____
_____

LUNCH

SNACK
_____
_____

DINNER

SNACK
_____
_____

MEDICATION

FOOD TRIALING: _____ DAYS TRIALED: _____

SYMPTOMS

		X	NOTES/TIME STARTED	NOTES
SKIN	ITCHINESS			
	HIVES			
	RASH			
	SWELLING			
	REDNESS			
	PALENESS			
	ECZEMA			
	OTHER			
THROAT / STOMACH	DIFFICULTY SWALLOWING			
	CHOKING			
	REFLUX			
	IMMEDIATE VOMITING			
	DELAYED VOMITING			
	OTHER			
NASAL / SINUSES	STUFFY NOSE			
	RUNNY NOSE			
	ITCHY THROAT			
	HOARSE VOICE			
	REPETITIVE COUGHING			
	OTHER			
LUNGS	WHEEZING			
	SHORTNESS OF BREATH			
	DIFFICULTY BREATHING			
	OTHER			
STOOL	DIARRHEA			
	CONSTIPATION			
	BLOODY STOOL			
	MUCOUS IN STOOL			
	GREEN STOOL			
	UNUSUAL ODOR			
	OTHER			
NEUROLOGICAL	IRRITABILITY			
	HYPERACTIVITY			
	INCREASED TANTRUMS			
	CLINGINESS			
	FAINTING			
	DIZZINESS			
	EXCESSIVE CRYING			
	LETHARGY/FATIGUE			
	MOTOR TICS			
	SEIZURES			
	DIFFICULTY SLEEPING			
	FEVER			
	LOW TEMPERATURE			
	OTHER			

DATE _____

MOM'S MEALS

BREAKFAST

SNACK

LUNCH

SNACK

DINNER

SNACK

MEDICATION

CHILD'S MEALS

BREAKFAST

SNACK

LUNCH

SNACK

DINNER

SNACK

MEDICATION

FOOD TRIALING: _____   DAYS TRIALED: _____

SYMPTOMS

		X	NOTES/TIME STARTED	NOTES

	Symptom	X	NOTES/TIME STARTED	NOTES
SKIN	ITCHINESS			
	HIVES			
	RASH			
	SWELLING			
	REDNESS			
	PALENESS			
	ECZEMA			
	OTHER			
THROAT / STOMACH	DIFFICULTY SWALLOWING			
	CHOKING			
	REFLUX			
	IMMEDIATE VOMITING			
	DELAYED VOMITING			
	OTHER			
NASAL / SINUSES	STUFFY NOSE			
	RUNNY NOSE			
	ITCHY THROAT			
	HOARSE VOICE			
	REPETITIVE COUGHING			
	OTHER			
LUNGS	WHEEZING			
	SHORTNESS OF BREATH			
	DIFFICULTY BREATHING			
	OTHER			
STOOL	DIARRHEA			
	CONSTIPATION			
	BLOODY STOOL			
	MUCOUS IN STOOL			
	GREEN STOOL			
	UNUSUAL ODOR			
	OTHER			
NEUROLOGICAL	IRRITABILITY			
	HYPERACTIVITY			
	INCREASED TANTRUMS			
	CLINGINESS			
	FAINTING			
	DIZZINESS			
	EXCESSIVE CRYING			
	LETHARGY/FATIGUE			
	MOTOR TICS			
	SEIZURES			
	DIFFICULTY SLEEPING			
	FEVER			
	LOW TEMPERATURE			
	OTHER			

DATE _____

MOM'S MEALS
BREAKFAST

SNACK
_____

LUNCH

SNACK
_____

DINNER

SNACK
_____

MEDICATION

CHILD'S MEALS
BREAKFAST

SNACK
_____

LUNCH

SNACK
_____

DINNER

SNACK
_____

MEDICATION

FOOD TRIALING: _____ DAYS TRIALED: _____

SYMPTOMS

		X	NOTES/TIME STARTED	NOTES

		X	NOTES/TIME STARTED	NOTES
SKIN	ITCHINESS			
	HIVES			
	RASH			
	SWELLING			
	REDNESS			
	PALENESS			
	ECZEMA			
	OTHER			
THROAT STOMACH	DIFFICULTY SWALLOWING			
	CHOKING			
	REFLUX			
	IMMEDIATE VOMITING			
	DELAYED VOMITING			
	OTHER			
NASAL SINUSES	STUFFY NOSE			
	RUNNY NOSE			
	ITCHY THROAT			
	HOARSE VOICE			
	REPETITIVE COUGHING			
	OTHER			
LUNGS	WHEEZING			
	SHORTNESS OF BREATH			
	DIFFICULTY BREATHING			
	OTHER			
STOOL	DIARRHEA			
	CONSTIPATION			
	BLOODY STOOL			
	MUCOUS IN STOOL			
	GREEN STOOL			
	UNUSUAL ODOR			
	OTHER			
NEUROLOGICAL	IRRITABILITY			
	HYPERACTIVITY			
	INCREASED TANTRUMS			
	CLINGINESS			
	FAINTING			
	DIZZINESS			
	EXCESSIVE CRYING			
	LETHARGY/FATIGUE			
	MOTOR TICS			
	SEIZURES			
	DIFFICULTY SLEEPING			
	FEVER			
	LOW TEMPERATURE			
	OTHER			

DATE _____

MOM'S MEALS
BREAKFAST

SNACK

LUNCH

SNACK

DINNER

SNACK

MEDICATION

CHILD'S MEALS
BREAKFAST

SNACK

LUNCH

SNACK

DINNER

SNACK

MEDICATION

FOOD TRIALING: _____ DAYS TRIALED: _____

SYMPTOMS

		X	NOTES/TIME STARTED	NOTES
SKIN	ITCHINESS			
	HIVES			
	RASH			
	SWELLING			
	REDNESS			
	PALENESS			
	ECZEMA			
	OTHER			
THROAT STOMACH	DIFFICULTY SWALLOWING			
	CHOKING			
	REFLUX			
	IMMEDIATE VOMITING			
	DELAYED VOMITING			
	OTHER			
NASAL SINUSES	STUFFY NOSE			
	RUNNY NOSE			
	ITCHY THROAT			
	HOARSE VOICE			
	REPETITIVE COUGHING			
	OTHER			
LUNGS	WHEEZING			
	SHORTNESS OF BREATH			
	DIFFICULTY BREATHING			
	OTHER			
STOOL	DIARRHEA			
	CONSTIPATION			
	BLOODY STOOL			
	MUCOUS IN STOOL			
	GREEN STOOL			
	UNUSUAL ODOR			
	OTHER			
NEUROLOGICAL	IRRITABILITY			
	HYPERACTIVITY			
	INCREASED TANTRUMS			
	CLINGINESS			
	FAINTING			
	DIZZINESS			
	EXCESSIVE CRYING			
	LETHARGY/FATIGUE			
	MOTOR TICS			
	SEIZURES			
	DIFFICULTY SLEEPING			
	FEVER			
	LOW TEMPERATURE			
	OTHER			

DATE _____

MOM'S MEALS

BREAKFAST

SNACK

LUNCH

SNACK

DINNER

SNACK

MEDICATION

CHILD'S MEALS

BREAKFAST

SNACK

LUNCH

SNACK

DINNER

SNACK

MEDICATION

FOOD TRIALING: _____ DAYS TRIALED: _____

SYMPTOMS

		X	NOTES/TIME STARTED	NOTES
SKIN	ITCHINESS			
	HIVES			
	RASH			
	SWELLING			
	REDNESS			
	PALENESS			
	ECZEMA			
	OTHER			
THROAT STOMACH	DIFFICULTY SWALLOWING			
	CHOKING			
	REFLUX			
	IMMEDIATE VOMITING			
	DELAYED VOMITING			
	OTHER			
NASAL SINUSES	STUFFY NOSE			
	RUNNY NOSE			
	ITCHY THROAT			
	HOARSE VOICE			
	REPETITIVE COUGHING			
	OTHER			
LUNGS	WHEEZING			
	SHORTNESS OF BREATH			
	DIFFICULTY BREATHING			
	OTHER			
STOOL	DIARRHEA			
	CONSTIPATION			
	BLOODY STOOL			
	MUCOUS IN STOOL			
	GREEN STOOL			
	UNUSUAL ODOR			
	OTHER			
NEUROLOGICAL	IRRITABILITY			
	HYPERACTIVITY			
	INCREASED TANTRUMS			
	CLINGINESS			
	FAINTING			
	DIZZINESS			
	EXCESSIVE CRYING			
	LETHARGY/FATIGUE			
	MOTOR TICS			
	SEIZURES			
	DIFFICULTY SLEEPING			
	FEVER			
	LOW TEMPERATURE			
	OTHER			

DATE _____

MOM'S MEALS

BREAKFAST

SNACK

LUNCH

SNACK

DINNER

SNACK

MEDICATION

CHILD'S MEALS

BREAKFAST

SNACK

LUNCH

SNACK

DINNER

SNACK

MEDICATION

FOOD TRIALING: _____ DAYS TRIALED: _____

SYMPTOMS

		X	NOTES/TIME STARTED	NOTES
SKIN	ITCHINESS			
	HIVES			
	RASH			
	SWELLING			
	REDNESS			
	PALENESS			
	ECZEMA			
	OTHER			
THROAT STOMACH	DIFFICULTY SWALLOWING			
	CHOKING			
	REFLUX			
	IMMEDIATE VOMITING			
	DELAYED VOMITING			
	OTHER			
NASAL SINUSES	STUFFY NOSE			
	RUNNY NOSE			
	ITCHY THROAT			
	HOARSE VOICE			
	REPETITIVE COUGHING			
	OTHER			
LUNGS	WHEEZING			
	SHORTNESS OF BREATH			
	DIFFICULTY BREATHING			
	OTHER			
STOOL	DIARRHEA			
	CONSTIPATION			
	BLOODY STOOL			
	MUCOUS IN STOOL			
	GREEN STOOL			
	UNUSUAL ODOR			
	OTHER			
NEUROLOGICAL	IRRITABILITY			
	HYPERACTIVITY			
	INCREASED TANTRUMS			
	CLINGINESS			
	FAINTING			
	DIZZINESS			
	EXCESSIVE CRYING			
	LETHARGY/FATIGUE			
	MOTOR TICS			
	SEIZURES			
	DIFFICULTY SLEEPING			
	FEVER			
	LOW TEMPERATURE			
	OTHER			

DATE _____

MOM'S MEALS
BREAKFAST

SNACK
_____
_____
_____

LUNCH

SNACK
_____
_____
_____

DINNER

SNACK
_____
_____
_____

MEDICATION

CHILD'S MEALS
BREAKFAST

SNACK
_____
_____
_____

LUNCH

SNACK
_____
_____
_____

DINNER

SNACK
_____
_____
_____

MEDICATION

FOOD TRIALING: _____   DAYS TRIALED: _____

SYMPTOMS

		X	NOTES/TIME STARTED	NOTES

		X	NOTES/TIME STARTED	NOTES
SKIN	ITCHINESS			
	HIVES			
	RASH			
	SWELLING			
	REDNESS			
	PALENESS			
	ECZEMA			
	OTHER			
THROAT / STOMACH	DIFFICULTY SWALLOWING			
	CHOKING			
	REFLUX			
	IMMEDIATE VOMITING			
	DELAYED VOMITING			
	OTHER			
NASAL / SINUSES	STUFFY NOSE			
	RUNNY NOSE			
	ITCHY THROAT			
	HOARSE VOICE			
	REPETITIVE COUGHING			
	OTHER			
LUNGS	WHEEZING			
	SHORTNESS OF BREATH			
	DIFFICULTY BREATHING			
	OTHER			
STOOL	DIARRHEA			
	CONSTIPATION			
	BLOODY STOOL			
	MUCOUS IN STOOL			
	GREEN STOOL			
	UNUSUAL ODOR			
	OTHER			
NEUROLOGICAL	IRRITABILITY			
	HYPERACTIVITY			
	INCREASED TANTRUMS			
	CLINGINESS			
	FAINTING			
	DIZZINESS			
	EXCESSIVE CRYING			
	LETHARGY/FATIGUE			
	MOTOR TICS			
	SEIZURES			
	DIFFICULTY SLEEPING			
	FEVER			
	LOW TEMPERATURE			
	OTHER			

DATE _____

MOM'S MEALS
BREAKFAST

SNACK

LUNCH

SNACK

DINNER

SNACK

MEDICATION

CHILD'S MEALS
BREAKFAST

SNACK

LUNCH

SNACK

DINNER

SNACK

MEDICATION

FOOD TRIALING: _____ DAYS TRIALED: _____

SYMPTOMS

		X	NOTES/TIME STARTED	NOTES

		X	NOTES/TIME STARTED	NOTES
SKIN	ITCHINESS			
	HIVES			
	RASH			
	SWELLING			
	REDNESS			
	PALENESS			
	ECZEMA			
	OTHER			
THROAT STOMACH	DIFFICULTY SWALLOWING			
	CHOKING			
	REFLUX			
	IMMEDIATE VOMITING			
	DELAYED VOMITING			
	OTHER			
NASAL SINUSES	STUFFY NOSE			
	RUNNY NOSE			
	ITCHY THROAT			
	HOARSE VOICE			
	REPETITIVE COUGHING			
	OTHER			
LUNGS	WHEEZING			
	SHORTNESS OF BREATH			
	DIFFICULTY BREATHING			
	OTHER			
STOOL	DIARRHEA			
	CONSTIPATION			
	BLOODY STOOL			
	MUCOUS IN STOOL			
	GREEN STOOL			
	UNUSUAL ODOR			
	OTHER			
NEUROLOGICAL	IRRITABILITY			
	HYPERACTIVITY			
	INCREASED TANTRUMS			
	CLINGINESS			
	FAINTING			
	DIZZINESS			
	EXCESSIVE CRYING			
	LETHARGY/FATIGUE			
	MOTOR TICS			
	SEIZURES			
	DIFFICULTY SLEEPING			
	FEVER			
	LOW TEMPERATURE			
	OTHER			

DATE _____

MOM'S MEALS

BREAKFAST

SNACK

LUNCH

SNACK

DINNER

SNACK

MEDICATION

CHILD'S MEALS

BREAKFAST

SNACK

LUNCH

SNACK

DINNER

SNACK

MEDICATION

FOOD TRIALING: _____ DAYS TRIALED: _____

SYMPTOMS

	Symptom	X	NOTES/TIME STARTED	NOTES
SKIN	ITCHINESS			
	HIVES			
	RASH			
	SWELLING			
	REDNESS			
	PALENESS			
	ECZEMA			
	OTHER			
THROAT / STOMACH	DIFFICULTY SWALLOWING			
	CHOKING			
	REFLUX			
	IMMEDIATE VOMITING			
	DELAYED VOMITING			
	OTHER			
NASAL / SINUSES	STUFFY NOSE			
	RUNNY NOSE			
	ITCHY THROAT			
	HOARSE VOICE			
	REPETITIVE COUGHING			
	OTHER			
LUNGS	WHEEZING			
	SHORTNESS OF BREATH			
	DIFFICULTY BREATHING			
	OTHER			
STOOL	DIARRHEA			
	CONSTIPATION			
	BLOODY STOOL			
	MUCOUS IN STOOL			
	GREEN STOOL			
	UNUSUAL ODOR			
	OTHER			
NEUROLOGICAL	IRRITABILITY			
	HYPERACTIVITY			
	INCREASED TANTRUMS			
	CLINGINESS			
	FAINTING			
	DIZZINESS			
	EXCESSIVE CRYING			
	LETHARGY/FATIGUE			
	MOTOR TICS			
	SEIZURES			
	DIFFICULTY SLEEPING			
	FEVER			
	LOW TEMPERATURE			
	OTHER			

DATE _____

MOM'S MEALS

BREAKFAST

SNACK

LUNCH

SNACK

DINNER

SNACK

MEDICATION

CHILD'S MEALS

BREAKFAST

SNACK

LUNCH

SNACK

DINNER

SNACK

MEDICATION

FOOD TRIALING: _____   DAYS TRIALED: _____

SYMPTOMS

		X	NOTES/TIME STARTED	NOTES
SKIN	ITCHINESS			
	HIVES			
	RASH			
	SWELLING			
	REDNESS			
	PALENESS			
	ECZEMA			
	OTHER			
THROAT STOMACH	DIFFICULTY SWALLOWING			
	CHOKING			
	REFLUX			
	IMMEDIATE VOMITING			
	DELAYED VOMITING			
	OTHER			
NASAL SINUSES	STUFFY NOSE			
	RUNNY NOSE			
	ITCHY THROAT			
	HOARSE VOICE			
	REPETITIVE COUGHING			
	OTHER			
LUNGS	WHEEZING			
	SHORTNESS OF BREATH			
	DIFFICULTY BREATHING			
	OTHER			
STOOL	DIARRHEA			
	CONSTIPATION			
	BLOODY STOOL			
	MUCOUS IN STOOL			
	GREEN STOOL			
	UNUSUAL ODOR			
	OTHER			
NEUROLOGICAL	IRRITABILITY			
	HYPERACTIVITY			
	INCREASED TANTRUMS			
	CLINGINESS			
	FAINTING			
	DIZZINESS			
	EXCESSIVE CRYING			
	LETHARGY/FATIGUE			
	MOTOR TICS			
	SEIZURES			
	DIFFICULTY SLEEPING			
	FEVER			
	LOW TEMPERATURE			
	OTHER			

DATE _____

MOM'S MEALS
BREAKFAST

SNACK

LUNCH

SNACK

DINNER

SNACK

MEDICATION

CHILD'S MEALS
BREAKFAST

SNACK

LUNCH

SNACK

DINNER

SNACK

MEDICATION

FOOD TRIALING: _____   DAYS TRIALED: _____

SYMPTOMS

		X	NOTES/TIME STARTED	NOTES

	Symptom	X	NOTES/TIME STARTED	NOTES
SKIN	ITCHINESS			
	HIVES			
	RASH			
	SWELLING			
	REDNESS			
	PALENESS			
	ECZEMA			
	OTHER			
THROAT / STOMACH	DIFFICULTY SWALLOWING			
	CHOKING			
	REFLUX			
	IMMEDIATE VOMITING			
	DELAYED VOMITING			
	OTHER			
NASAL / SINUSES	STUFFY NOSE			
	RUNNY NOSE			
	ITCHY THROAT			
	HOARSE VOICE			
	REPETITIVE COUGHING			
	OTHER			
LUNGS	WHEEZING			
	SHORTNESS OF BREATH			
	DIFFICULTY BREATHING			
	OTHER			
STOOL	DIARRHEA			
	CONSTIPATION			
	BLOODY STOOL			
	MUCOUS IN STOOL			
	GREEN STOOL			
	UNUSUAL ODOR			
	OTHER			
NEUROLOGICAL	IRRITABILITY			
	HYPERACTIVITY			
	INCREASED TANTRUMS			
	CLINGINESS			
	FAINTING			
	DIZZINESS			
	EXCESSIVE CRYING			
	LETHARGY/FATIGUE			
	MOTOR TICS			
	SEIZURES			
	DIFFICULTY SLEEPING			
	FEVER			
	LOW TEMPERATURE			
	OTHER			

DATE_____

MOM'S MEALS

BREAKFAST

SNACK

LUNCH

SNACK

DINNER

SNACK

MEDICATION

CHILD'S MEALS

BREAKFAST

SNACK

LUNCH

SNACK

DINNER

SNACK

MEDICATION

FOOD TRIALING: _____ DAYS TRIALED: _____

SYMPTOMS

	Symptom	X	NOTES/TIME STARTED	NOTES
SKIN	ITCHINESS			
	HIVES			
	RASH			
	SWELLING			
	REDNESS			
	PALENESS			
	ECZEMA			
	OTHER			
THROAT / STOMACH	DIFFICULTY SWALLOWING			
	CHOKING			
	REFLUX			
	IMMEDIATE VOMITING			
	DELAYED VOMITING			
	OTHER			
NASAL / SINUSES	STUFFY NOSE			
	RUNNY NOSE			
	ITCHY THROAT			
	HOARSE VOICE			
	REPETITIVE COUGHING			
	OTHER			
LUNGS	WHEEZING			
	SHORTNESS OF BREATH			
	DIFFICULTY BREATHING			
	OTHER			
STOOL	DIARRHEA			
	CONSTIPATION			
	BLOODY STOOL			
	MUCOUS IN STOOL			
	GREEN STOOL			
	UNUSUAL ODOR			
	OTHER			
NEUROLOGICAL	IRRITABILITY			
	HYPERACTIVITY			
	INCREASED TANTRUMS			
	CLINGINESS			
	FAINTING			
	DIZZINESS			
	EXCESSIVE CRYING			
	LETHARGY/FATIGUE			
	MOTOR TICS			
	SEIZURES			
	DIFFICULTY SLEEPING			
	FEVER			
	LOW TEMPERATURE			
	OTHER			

DATE _____

MOM'S MEALS
BREAKFAST

SNACK
_____
_____
_____

LUNCH

SNACK
_____
_____
_____

DINNER

SNACK
_____

MEDICATION

CHILD'S MEALS
BREAKFAST

SNACK
_____
_____
_____

LUNCH

SNACK
_____
_____
_____

DINNER

SNACK
_____

MEDICATION

FOOD TRIALING: _____   DAYS TRIALED: _____

SYMPTOMS

		X	NOTES/TIME STARTED	NOTES

	SYMPTOM	X	NOTES/TIME STARTED	NOTES
SKIN	ITCHINESS			
	HIVES			
	RASH			
	SWELLING			
	REDNESS			
	PALENESS			
	ECZEMA			
	OTHER			
THROAT STOMACH	DIFFICULTY SWALLOWING			
	CHOKING			
	REFLUX			
	IMMEDIATE VOMITING			
	DELAYED VOMITING			
	OTHER			
NASAL SINUSES	STUFFY NOSE			
	RUNNY NOSE			
	ITCHY THROAT			
	HOARSE VOICE			
	REPETITIVE COUGHING			
	OTHER			
LUNGS	WHEEZING			
	SHORTNESS OF BREATH			
	DIFFICULTY BREATHING			
	OTHER			
STOOL	DIARRHEA			
	CONSTIPATION			
	BLOODY STOOL			
	MUCOUS IN STOOL			
	GREEN STOOL			
	UNUSUAL ODOR			
	OTHER			
NEUROLOGICAL	IRRITABILITY			
	HYPERACTIVITY			
	INCREASED TANTRUMS			
	CLINGINESS			
	FAINTING			
	DIZZINESS			
	EXCESSIVE CRYING			
	LETHARGY/FATIGUE			
	MOTOR TICS			
	SEIZURES			
	DIFFICULTY SLEEPING			
	FEVER			
	LOW TEMPERATURE			
	OTHER			

DATE _____

MOM'S MEALS

BREAKFAST

SNACK

LUNCH

SNACK

DINNER

SNACK

MEDICATION

CHILD'S MEALS

BREAKFAST

SNACK

LUNCH

SNACK

DINNER

SNACK

MEDICATION

FOOD TRIALING: _____ DAYS TRIALED: _____

SYMPTOMS

		X	NOTES/TIME STARTED	NOTES
SKIN	ITCHINESS			
	HIVES			
	RASH			
	SWELLING			
	REDNESS			
	PALENESS			
	ECZEMA			
	OTHER			
THROAT STOMACH	DIFFICULTY SWALLOWING			
	CHOKING			
	REFLUX			
	IMMEDIATE VOMITING			
	DELAYED VOMITING			
	OTHER			
NASAL SINUSES	STUFFY NOSE			
	RUNNY NOSE			
	ITCHY THROAT			
	HOARSE VOICE			
	REPETITIVE COUGHING			
	OTHER			
LUNGS	WHEEZING			
	SHORTNESS OF BREATH			
	DIFFICULTY BREATHING			
	OTHER			
STOOL	DIARRHEA			
	CONSTIPATION			
	BLOODY STOOL			
	MUCOUS IN STOOL			
	GREEN STOOL			
	UNUSUAL ODOR			
	OTHER			
NEUROLOGICAL	IRRITABILITY			
	HYPERACTIVITY			
	INCREASED TANTRUMS			
	CLINGINESS			
	FAINTING			
	DIZZINESS			
	EXCESSIVE CRYING			
	LETHARGY/FATIGUE			
	MOTOR TICS			
	SEIZURES			
	DIFFICULTY SLEEPING			
	FEVER			
	LOW TEMPERATURE			
	OTHER			

DATE _____

MOM'S MEALS

BREAKFAST

SNACK

LUNCH

SNACK

DINNER

SNACK

MEDICATION

CHILD'S MEALS

BREAKFAST

SNACK

LUNCH

SNACK

DINNER

SNACK

MEDICATION

FOOD TRIALING: _____ DAYS TRIALED: _____

SYMPTOMS

		X	NOTES/TIME STARTED	NOTES
SKIN	ITCHINESS			
	HIVES			
	RASH			
	SWELLING			
	REDNESS			
	PALENESS			
	ECZEMA			
	OTHER			
THROAT STOMACH	DIFFICULTY SWALLOWING			
	CHOKING			
	REFLUX			
	IMMEDIATE VOMITING			
	DELAYED VOMITING			
	OTHER			
NASAL SINUSES	STUFFY NOSE			
	RUNNY NOSE			
	ITCHY THROAT			
	HOARSE VOICE			
	REPETITIVE COUGHING			
	OTHER			
LUNGS	WHEEZING			
	SHORTNESS OF BREATH			
	DIFFICULTY BREATHING			
	OTHER			
STOOL	DIARRHEA			
	CONSTIPATION			
	BLOODY STOOL			
	MUCOUS IN STOOL			
	GREEN STOOL			
	UNUSUAL ODOR			
	OTHER			
NEUROLOGICAL	IRRITABILITY			
	HYPERACTIVITY			
	INCREASED TANTRUMS			
	CLINGINESS			
	FAINTING			
	DIZZINESS			
	EXCESSIVE CRYING			
	LETHARGY/FATIGUE			
	MOTOR TICS			
	SEIZURES			
	DIFFICULTY SLEEPING			
	FEVER			
	LOW TEMPERATURE			
	OTHER			

DATE _____

MOM'S MEALS
BREAKFAST

SNACK
_____

LUNCH

SNACK
_____

DINNER

SNACK
_____

MEDICATION

CHILD'S MEALS
BREAKFAST

SNACK
_____

LUNCH

SNACK
_____

DINNER

SNACK
_____

MEDICATION

FOOD TRIALING: _____ DAYS TRIALED: _____

SYMPTOMS

		X	NOTES/TIME STARTED	NOTES
SKIN	ITCHINESS			
	HIVES			
	RASH			
	SWELLING			
	REDNESS			
	PALENESS			
	ECZEMA			
	OTHER			
THROAT STOMACH	DIFFICULTY SWALLOWING			
	CHOKING			
	REFLUX			
	IMMEDIATE VOMITING			
	DELAYED VOMITING			
	OTHER			
NASAL SINUSES	STUFFY NOSE			
	RUNNY NOSE			
	ITCHY THROAT			
	HOARSE VOICE			
	REPETITIVE COUGHING			
	OTHER			
LUNGS	WHEEZING			
	SHORTNESS OF BREATH			
	DIFFICULTY BREATHING			
	OTHER			
STOOL	DIARRHEA			
	CONSTIPATION			
	BLOODY STOOL			
	MUCOUS IN STOOL			
	GREEN STOOL			
	UNUSUAL ODOR			
	OTHER			
NEUROLOGICAL	IRRITABILITY			
	HYPERACTIVITY			
	INCREASED TANTRUMS			
	CLINGINESS			
	FAINTING			
	DIZZINESS			
	EXCESSIVE CRYING			
	LETHARGY/FATIGUE			
	MOTOR TICS			
	SEIZURES			
	DIFFICULTY SLEEPING			
	FEVER			
	LOW TEMPERATURE			
	OTHER			

DATE _____

MOM'S MEALS
BREAKFAST

SNACK
_____
_____
_____

LUNCH

SNACK
_____
_____
_____

DINNER

SNACK
_____
_____

MEDICATION

CHILD'S MEALS
BREAKFAST

SNACK
_____
_____
_____

LUNCH

SNACK
_____
_____
_____

DINNER

SNACK
_____
_____

MEDICATION

FOOD TRIALING: _____   DAYS TRIALED: _____

SYMPTOMS

	SYMPTOMS	X NOTES/TIME STARTED	NOTES
SKIN	ITCHINESS		
	HIVES		
	RASH		
	SWELLING		
	REDNESS		
	PALENESS		
	ECZEMA		
	OTHER		
THROAT STOMACH	DIFFICULTY SWALLOWING		
	CHOKING		
	REFLUX		
	IMMEDIATE VOMITING		
	DELAYED VOMITING		
	OTHER		
NASAL SINUSES	STUFFY NOSE		
	RUNNY NOSE		
	ITCHY THROAT		
	HOARSE VOICE		
	REPETITIVE COUGHING		
	OTHER		
LUNGS	WHEEZING		
	SHORTNESS OF BREATH		
	DIFFICULTY BREATHING		
	OTHER		
STOOL	DIARRHEA		
	CONSTIPATION		
	BLOODY STOOL		
	MUCOUS IN STOOL		
	GREEN STOOL		
	UNUSUAL ODOR		
	OTHER		
NEUROLOGICAL	IRRITABILITY		
	HYPERACTIVITY		
	INCREASED TANTRUMS		
	CLINGINESS		
	FAINTING		
	DIZZINESS		
	EXCESSIVE CRYING		
	LETHARGY/FATIGUE		
	MOTOR TICS		
	SEIZURES		
	DIFFICULTY SLEEPING		
	FEVER		
	LOW TEMPERATURE		
	OTHER		

DATE _____

MOM'S MEALS

BREAKFAST

SNACK

LUNCH

SNACK

DINNER

SNACK

MEDICATION

CHILD'S MEALS

BREAKFAST

SNACK

LUNCH

SNACK

DINNER

SNACK

MEDICATION

FOOD TRIALING: _____ DAYS TRIALED: _____

SYMPTOMS

		X	NOTES/TIME STARTED	NOTES
SKIN	ITCHINESS			
	HIVES			
	RASH			
	SWELLING			
	REDNESS			
	PALENESS			
	ECZEMA			
	OTHER			
THROAT / STOMACH	DIFFICULTY SWALLOWING			
	CHOKING			
	REFLUX			
	IMMEDIATE VOMITING			
	DELAYED VOMITING			
	OTHER			
NASAL / SINUSES	STUFFY NOSE			
	RUNNY NOSE			
	ITCHY THROAT			
	HOARSE VOICE			
	REPETITIVE COUGHING			
	OTHER			
LUNGS	WHEEZING			
	SHORTNESS OF BREATH			
	DIFFICULTY BREATHING			
	OTHER			
STOOL	DIARRHEA			
	CONSTIPATION			
	BLOODY STOOL			
	MUCOUS IN STOOL			
	GREEN STOOL			
	UNUSUAL ODOR			
	OTHER			
NEUROLOGICAL	IRRITABILITY			
	HYPERACTIVITY			
	INCREASED TANTRUMS			
	CLINGINESS			
	FAINTING			
	DIZZINESS			
	EXCESSIVE CRYING			
	LETHARGY/FATIGUE			
	MOTOR TICS			
	SEIZURES			
	DIFFICULTY SLEEPING			
	FEVER			
	LOW TEMPERATURE			
	OTHER			

DATE _____

MOM'S MEALS

BREAKFAST

SNACK

LUNCH

SNACK

DINNER

SNACK

MEDICATION

CHILD'S MEALS

BREAKFAST

SNACK

LUNCH

SNACK

DINNER

SNACK

MEDICATION

FOOD TRIALING: _____ DAYS TRIALED: _____

SYMPTOMS

		X	NOTES/TIME STARTED	NOTES
SKIN	ITCHINESS			
	HIVES			
	RASH			
	SWELLING			
	REDNESS			
	PALENESS			
	ECZEMA			
	OTHER			
THROAT STOMACH	DIFFICULTY SWALLOWING			
	CHOKING			
	REFLUX			
	IMMEDIATE VOMITING			
	DELAYED VOMITING			
	OTHER			
NASAL SINUSES	STUFFY NOSE			
	RUNNY NOSE			
	ITCHY THROAT			
	HOARSE VOICE			
	REPETITIVE COUGHING			
	OTHER			
LUNGS	WHEEZING			
	SHORTNESS OF BREATH			
	DIFFICULTY BREATHING			
	OTHER			
STOOL	DIARRHEA			
	CONSTIPATION			
	BLOODY STOOL			
	MUCOUS IN STOOL			
	GREEN STOOL			
	UNUSUAL ODOR			
	OTHER			
NEUROLOGICAL	IRRITABILITY			
	HYPERACTIVITY			
	INCREASED TANTRUMS			
	CLINGINESS			
	FAINTING			
	DIZZINESS			
	EXCESSIVE CRYING			
	LETHARGY/FATIGUE			
	MOTOR TICS			
	SEIZURES			
	DIFFICULTY SLEEPING			
	FEVER			
	LOW TEMPERATURE			
	OTHER			

DATE _____

MOM'S MEALS
BREAKFAST

SNACK

LUNCH

SNACK

DINNER

SNACK

MEDICATION

CHILD'S MEALS
BREAKFAST

SNACK

LUNCH

SNACK

DINNER

SNACK

MEDICATION

FOOD TRIALING: _____ DAYS TRIALED: _____

SYMPTOMS

		X	NOTES/TIME STARTED	NOTES
SKIN	ITCHINESS			
	HIVES			
	RASH			
	SWELLING			
	REDNESS			
	PALENESS			
	ECZEMA			
	OTHER			
THROAT STOMACH	DIFFICULTY SWALLOWING			
	CHOKING			
	REFLUX			
	IMMEDIATE VOMITING			
	DELAYED VOMITING			
	OTHER			
NASAL SINUSES	STUFFY NOSE			
	RUNNY NOSE			
	ITCHY THROAT			
	HOARSE VOICE			
	REPETITIVE COUGHING			
	OTHER			
LUNGS	WHEEZING			
	SHORTNESS OF BREATH			
	DIFFICULTY BREATHING			
	OTHER			
STOOL	DIARRHEA			
	CONSTIPATION			
	BLOODY STOOL			
	MUCOUS IN STOOL			
	GREEN STOOL			
	UNUSUAL ODOR			
	OTHER			
NEUROLOGICAL	IRRITABILITY			
	HYPERACTIVITY			
	INCREASED TANTRUMS			
	CLINGINESS			
	FAINTING			
	DIZZINESS			
	EXCESSIVE CRYING			
	LETHARGY/FATIGUE			
	MOTOR TICS			
	SEIZURES			
	DIFFICULTY SLEEPING			
	FEVER			
	LOW TEMPERATURE			
	OTHER			

DATE _____

MOM'S MEALS

BREAKFAST

SNACK

LUNCH

SNACK

DINNER

SNACK

MEDICATION

CHILD'S MEALS

BREAKFAST

SNACK

LUNCH

SNACK

DINNER

SNACK

MEDICATION

FOOD TRIALING: _____   DAYS TRIALED: _____

SYMPTOMS

	X	NOTES/TIME STARTED	NOTES

		X	NOTES/TIME STARTED	NOTES
SKIN	ITCHINESS			
	HIVES			
	RASH			
	SWELLING			
	REDNESS			
	PALENESS			
	ECZEMA			
	OTHER			
THROAT / STOMACH	DIFFICULTY SWALLOWING			
	CHOKING			
	REFLUX			
	IMMEDIATE VOMITING			
	DELAYED VOMITING			
	OTHER			
NASAL / SINUSES	STUFFY NOSE			
	RUNNY NOSE			
	ITCHY THROAT			
	HOARSE VOICE			
	REPETITIVE COUGHING			
	OTHER			
LUNGS	WHEEZING			
	SHORTNESS OF BREATH			
	DIFFICULTY BREATHING			
	OTHER			
STOOL	DIARRHEA			
	CONSTIPATION			
	BLOODY STOOL			
	MUCOUS IN STOOL			
	GREEN STOOL			
	UNUSUAL ODOR			
	OTHER			
NEUROLOGICAL	IRRITABILITY			
	HYPERACTIVITY			
	INCREASED TANTRUMS			
	CLINGINESS			
	FAINTING			
	DIZZINESS			
	EXCESSIVE CRYING			
	LETHARGY/FATIGUE			
	MOTOR TICS			
	SEIZURES			
	DIFFICULTY SLEEPING			
	FEVER			
	LOW TEMPERATURE			
	OTHER			

DATE _____

MOM'S MEALS

BREAKFAST

SNACK

LUNCH

SNACK

DINNER

SNACK

MEDICATION

CHILD'S MEALS

BREAKFAST

SNACK

LUNCH

SNACK

DINNER

SNACK

MEDICATION

FOOD TRIALING: _____ DAYS TRIALED: _____

SYMPTOMS

		X	NOTES/TIME STARTED	NOTES

		X	NOTES/TIME STARTED	NOTES
SKIN	ITCHINESS			
	HIVES			
	RASH			
	SWELLING			
	REDNESS			
	PALENESS			
	ECZEMA			
	OTHER			
THROAT STOMACH	DIFFICULTY SWALLOWING			
	CHOKING			
	REFLUX			
	IMMEDIATE VOMITING			
	DELAYED VOMITING			
	OTHER			
NASAL SINUSES	STUFFY NOSE			
	RUNNY NOSE			
	ITCHY THROAT			
	HOARSE VOICE			
	REPETITIVE COUGHING			
	OTHER			
LUNGS	WHEEZING			
	SHORTNESS OF BREATH			
	DIFFICULTY BREATHING			
	OTHER			
STOOL	DIARRHEA			
	CONSTIPATION			
	BLOODY STOOL			
	MUCOUS IN STOOL			
	GREEN STOOL			
	UNUSUAL ODOR			
	OTHER			
NEUROLOGICAL	IRRITABILITY			
	HYPERACTIVITY			
	INCREASED TANTRUMS			
	CLINGINESS			
	FAINTING			
	DIZZINESS			
	EXCESSIVE CRYING			
	LETHARGY/FATIGUE			
	MOTOR TICS			
	SEIZURES			
	DIFFICULTY SLEEPING			
	FEVER			
	LOW TEMPERATURE			
	OTHER			

DATE _____

MOM'S MEALS

BREAKFAST

SNACK

LUNCH

SNACK

DINNER

SNACK

MEDICATION

CHILD'S MEALS

BREAKFAST

SNACK

LUNCH

SNACK

DINNER

SNACK

MEDICATION

FOOD TRIALING: _____   DAYS TRIALED: _____

SYMPTOMS

	SYMPTOMS	X	NOTES/TIME STARTED	NOTES
SKIN	ITCHINESS			
	HIVES			
	RASH			
	SWELLING			
	REDNESS			
	PALENESS			
	ECZEMA			
	OTHER			
THROAT STOMACH	DIFFICULTY SWALLOWING			
	CHOKING			
	REFLUX			
	IMMEDIATE VOMITING			
	DELAYED VOMITING			
	OTHER			
NASAL SINUSES	STUFFY NOSE			
	RUNNY NOSE			
	ITCHY THROAT			
	HOARSE VOICE			
	REPETITIVE COUGHING			
	OTHER			
LUNGS	WHEEZING			
	SHORTNESS OF BREATH			
	DIFFICULTY BREATHING			
	OTHER			
STOOL	DIARRHEA			
	CONSTIPATION			
	BLOODY STOOL			
	MUCOUS IN STOOL			
	GREEN STOOL			
	UNUSUAL ODOR			
	OTHER			
NEUROLOGICAL	IRRITABILITY			
	HYPERACTIVITY			
	INCREASED TANTRUMS			
	CLINGINESS			
	FAINTING			
	DIZZINESS			
	EXCESSIVE CRYING			
	LETHARGY/FATIGUE			
	MOTOR TICS			
	SEIZURES			
	DIFFICULTY SLEEPING			
	FEVER			
	LOW TEMPERATURE			
	OTHER			

DATE _____

MOM'S MEALS

BREAKFAST

SNACK

LUNCH

SNACK

DINNER

SNACK

MEDICATION

CHILD'S MEALS

BREAKFAST

SNACK

LUNCH

SNACK

DINNER

SNACK

MEDICATION

FOOD TRIALING: _____   DAYS TRIALED: _____

SYMPTOMS

		X	NOTES/TIME STARTED	NOTES
SKIN	ITCHINESS			
	HIVES			
	RASH			
	SWELLING			
	REDNESS			
	PALENESS			
	ECZEMA			
	OTHER			
THROAT STOMACH	DIFFICULTY SWALLOWING			
	CHOKING			
	REFLUX			
	IMMEDIATE VOMITING			
	DELAYED VOMITING			
	OTHER			
NASAL SINUSES	STUFFY NOSE			
	RUNNY NOSE			
	ITCHY THROAT			
	HOARSE VOICE			
	REPETITIVE COUGHING			
	OTHER			
LUNGS	WHEEZING			
	SHORTNESS OF BREATH			
	DIFFICULTY BREATHING			
	OTHER			
STOOL	DIARRHEA			
	CONSTIPATION			
	BLOODY STOOL			
	MUCOUS IN STOOL			
	GREEN STOOL			
	UNUSUAL ODOR			
	OTHER			
NEUROLOGICAL	IRRITABILITY			
	HYPERACTIVITY			
	INCREASED TANTRUMS			
	CLINGINESS			
	FAINTING			
	DIZZINESS			
	EXCESSIVE CRYING			
	LETHARGY/FATIGUE			
	MOTOR TICS			
	SEIZURES			
	DIFFICULTY SLEEPING			
	FEVER			
	LOW TEMPERATURE			
	OTHER			

DATE _____

MOM'S MEALS
BREAKFAST

SNACK
_____

LUNCH

SNACK
_____

DINNER

SNACK
_____

MEDICATION

CHILD'S MEALS
BREAKFAST

SNACK
_____

LUNCH

SNACK
_____

DINNER

SNACK
_____

MEDICATION

FOOD TRIALING: _____ DAYS TRIALED: _____

SYMPTOMS

		X	NOTES/TIME STARTED	NOTES

SKIN	ITCHINESS			
	HIVES			
	RASH			
	SWELLING			
	REDNESS			
	PALENESS			
	ECZEMA			
	OTHER			
THROAT STOMACH	DIFFICULTY SWALLOWING			
	CHOKING			
	REFLUX			
	IMMEDIATE VOMITING			
	DELAYED VOMITING			
	OTHER			
NASAL SINUSES	STUFFY NOSE			
	RUNNY NOSE			
	ITCHY THROAT			
	HOARSE VOICE			
	REPETITIVE COUGHING			
	OTHER			
LUNGS	WHEEZING			
	SHORTNESS OF BREATH			
	DIFFICULTY BREATHING			
	OTHER			
STOOL	DIARRHEA			
	CONSTIPATION			
	BLOODY STOOL			
	MUCOUS IN STOOL			
	GREEN STOOL			
	UNUSUAL ODOR			
	OTHER			
NEUROLOGICAL	IRRITABILITY			
	HYPERACTIVITY			
	INCREASED TANTRUMS			
	CLINGINESS			
	FAINTING			
	DIZZINESS			
	EXCESSIVE CRYING			
	LETHARGY/FATIGUE			
	MOTOR TICS			
	SEIZURES			
	DIFFICULTY SLEEPING			
	FEVER			
	LOW TEMPERATURE			
	OTHER			

DATE _____

MOM'S MEALS
BREAKFAST

SNACK

LUNCH

SNACK

DINNER

SNACK

MEDICATION

CHILD'S MEALS
BREAKFAST

SNACK

LUNCH

SNACK

DINNER

SNACK

MEDICATION

FOOD TRIALING: _____ DAYS TRIALED: _____

SYMPTOMS

	Symptom	X	NOTES/TIME STARTED	NOTES
SKIN	ITCHINESS			
	HIVES			
	RASH			
	SWELLING			
	REDNESS			
	PALENESS			
	ECZEMA			
	OTHER			
THROAT STOMACH	DIFFICULTY SWALLOWING			
	CHOKING			
	REFLUX			
	IMMEDIATE VOMITING			
	DELAYED VOMITING			
	OTHER			
NASAL SINUSES	STUFFY NOSE			
	RUNNY NOSE			
	ITCHY THROAT			
	HOARSE VOICE			
	REPETITIVE COUGHING			
	OTHER			
LUNGS	WHEEZING			
	SHORTNESS OF BREATH			
	DIFFICULTY BREATHING			
	OTHER			
STOOL	DIARRHEA			
	CONSTIPATION			
	BLOODY STOOL			
	MUCOUS IN STOOL			
	GREEN STOOL			
	UNUSUAL ODOR			
	OTHER			
NEUROLOGICAL	IRRITABILITY			
	HYPERACTIVITY			
	INCREASED TANTRUMS			
	CLINGINESS			
	FAINTING			
	DIZZINESS			
	EXCESSIVE CRYING			
	LETHARGY/FATIGUE			
	MOTOR TICS			
	SEIZURES			
	DIFFICULTY SLEEPING			
	FEVER			
	LOW TEMPERATURE			
	OTHER			

DATE _____

MOM'S MEALS

BREAKFAST

SNACK

LUNCH

SNACK

DINNER

SNACK

MEDICATION

CHILD'S MEALS

BREAKFAST

SNACK

LUNCH

SNACK

DINNER

SNACK

MEDICATION

FOOD TRIALING: _____ DAYS TRIALED: _____

SYMPTOMS

	SYMPTOMS	X	NOTES/TIME STARTED	NOTES
SKIN	ITCHINESS			
	HIVES			
	RASH			
	SWELLING			
	REDNESS			
	PALENESS			
	ECZEMA			
	OTHER			
THROAT STOMACH	DIFFICULTY SWALLOWING			
	CHOKING			
	REFLUX			
	IMMEDIATE VOMITING			
	DELAYED VOMITING			
	OTHER			
NASAL SINUSES	STUFFY NOSE			
	RUNNY NOSE			
	ITCHY THROAT			
	HOARSE VOICE			
	REPETITIVE COUGHING			
	OTHER			
LUNGS	WHEEZING			
	SHORTNESS OF BREATH			
	DIFFICULTY BREATHING			
	OTHER			
STOOL	DIARRHEA			
	CONSTIPATION			
	BLOODY STOOL			
	MUCOUS IN STOOL			
	GREEN STOOL			
	UNUSUAL ODOR			
	OTHER			
NEUROLOGICAL	IRRITABILITY			
	HYPERACTIVITY			
	INCREASED TANTRUMS			
	CLINGINESS			
	FAINTING			
	DIZZINESS			
	EXCESSIVE CRYING			
	LETHARGY/FATIGUE			
	MOTOR TICS			
	SEIZURES			
	DIFFICULTY SLEEPING			
	FEVER			
	LOW TEMPERATURE			
	OTHER			

DATE _____

MOM'S MEALS

BREAKFAST

SNACK

LUNCH

SNACK

DINNER

SNACK

MEDICATION

CHILD'S MEALS

BREAKFAST

SNACK

LUNCH

SNACK

DINNER

SNACK

MEDICATION

FOOD TRIALING: _____   DAYS TRIALED: _____

SYMPTOMS

		X	NOTES/TIME STARTED	NOTES

		X	NOTES/TIME STARTED	NOTES
SKIN	ITCHINESS			
	HIVES			
	RASH			
	SWELLING			
	REDNESS			
	PALENESS			
	ECZEMA			
	OTHER			
THROAT STOMACH	DIFFICULTY SWALLOWING			
	CHOKING			
	REFLUX			
	IMMEDIATE VOMITING			
	DELAYED VOMITING			
	OTHER			
NASAL SINUSES	STUFFY NOSE			
	RUNNY NOSE			
	ITCHY THROAT			
	HOARSE VOICE			
	REPETITIVE COUGHING			
	OTHER			
LUNGS	WHEEZING			
	SHORTNESS OF BREATH			
	DIFFICULTY BREATHING			
	OTHER			
STOOL	DIARRHEA			
	CONSTIPATION			
	BLOODY STOOL			
	MUCOUS IN STOOL			
	GREEN STOOL			
	UNUSUAL ODOR			
	OTHER			
NEUROLOGICAL	IRRITABILITY			
	HYPERACTIVITY			
	INCREASED TANTRUMS			
	CLINGINESS			
	FAINTING			
	DIZZINESS			
	EXCESSIVE CRYING			
	LETHARGY/FATIGUE			
	MOTOR TICS			
	SEIZURES			
	DIFFICULTY SLEEPING			
	FEVER			
	LOW TEMPERATURE			
	OTHER			

DATE _____

MOM'S MEALS

BREAKFAST

SNACK
_____
_____

LUNCH

SNACK
_____
_____

DINNER

SNACK
_____
_____

MEDICATION

CHILD'S MEALS

BREAKFAST

SNACK
_____
_____

LUNCH

SNACK
_____
_____

DINNER

SNACK
_____
_____

MEDICATION

FOOD TRIALING: _____   DAYS TRIALED: _____

SYMPTOMS

		X	NOTES/TIME STARTED	NOTES
SKIN	ITCHINESS			
	HIVES			
	RASH			
	SWELLING			
	REDNESS			
	PALENESS			
	ECZEMA			
	OTHER			
THROAT STOMACH	DIFFICULTY SWALLOWING			
	CHOKING			
	REFLUX			
	IMMEDIATE VOMITING			
	DELAYED VOMITING			
	OTHER			
NASAL SINUSES	STUFFY NOSE			
	RUNNY NOSE			
	ITCHY THROAT			
	HOARSE VOICE			
	REPETITIVE COUGHING			
	OTHER			
LUNGS	WHEEZING			
	SHORTNESS OF BREATH			
	DIFFICULTY BREATHING			
	OTHER			
STOOL	DIARRHEA			
	CONSTIPATION			
	BLOODY STOOL			
	MUCOUS IN STOOL			
	GREEN STOOL			
	UNUSUAL ODOR			
	OTHER			
NEUROLOGICAL	IRRITABILITY			
	HYPERACTIVITY			
	INCREASED TANTRUMS			
	CLINGINESS			
	FAINTING			
	DIZZINESS			
	EXCESSIVE CRYING			
	LETHARGY/FATIGUE			
	MOTOR TICS			
	SEIZURES			
	DIFFICULTY SLEEPING			
	FEVER			
	LOW TEMPERATURE			
	OTHER			

DATE _____

MOM'S MEALS

BREAKFAST

SNACK

LUNCH

SNACK

DINNER

SNACK

MEDICATION

CHILD'S MEALS

BREAKFAST

SNACK

LUNCH

SNACK

DINNER

SNACK

MEDICATION

FOOD TRIALING: _____ DAYS TRIALED: _____

SYMPTOMS

	Symptom	X NOTES/TIME STARTED	NOTES
SKIN	ITCHINESS		
	HIVES		
	RASH		
	SWELLING		
	REDNESS		
	PALENESS		
	ECZEMA		
	OTHER		
THROAT STOMACH	DIFFICULTY SWALLOWING		
	CHOKING		
	REFLUX		
	IMMEDIATE VOMITING		
	DELAYED VOMITING		
	OTHER		
NASAL SINUSES	STUFFY NOSE		
	RUNNY NOSE		
	ITCHY THROAT		
	HOARSE VOICE		
	REPETITIVE COUGHING		
	OTHER		
LUNGS	WHEEZING		
	SHORTNESS OF BREATH		
	DIFFICULTY BREATHING		
	OTHER		
STOOL	DIARRHEA		
	CONSTIPATION		
	BLOODY STOOL		
	MUCOUS IN STOOL		
	GREEN STOOL		
	UNUSUAL ODOR		
	OTHER		
NEUROLOGICAL	IRRITABILITY		
	HYPERACTIVITY		
	INCREASED TANTRUMS		
	CLINGINESS		
	FAINTING		
	DIZZINESS		
	EXCESSIVE CRYING		
	LETHARGY/FATIGUE		
	MOTOR TICS		
	SEIZURES		
	DIFFICULTY SLEEPING		
	FEVER		
	LOW TEMPERATURE		
	OTHER		

DATE _____

MOM'S MEALS

BREAKFAST

SNACK

LUNCH

SNACK

DINNER

SNACK

MEDICATION

CHILD'S MEALS

BREAKFAST

SNACK

LUNCH

SNACK

DINNER

SNACK

MEDICATION

FOOD TRIALING: _____   DAYS TRIALED: _____

SYMPTOMS

		X	NOTES/TIME STARTED	NOTES

	SYMPTOM	X	NOTES/TIME STARTED	NOTES
SKIN	ITCHINESS			
	HIVES			
	RASH			
	SWELLING			
	REDNESS			
	PALENESS			
	ECZEMA			
	OTHER			
THROAT / STOMACH	DIFFICULTY SWALLOWING			
	CHOKING			
	REFLUX			
	IMMEDIATE VOMITING			
	DELAYED VOMITING			
	OTHER			
NASAL / SINUSES	STUFFY NOSE			
	RUNNY NOSE			
	ITCHY THROAT			
	HOARSE VOICE			
	REPETITIVE COUGHING			
	OTHER			
LUNGS	WHEEZING			
	SHORTNESS OF BREATH			
	DIFFICULTY BREATHING			
	OTHER			
STOOL	DIARRHEA			
	CONSTIPATION			
	BLOODY STOOL			
	MUCOUS IN STOOL			
	GREEN STOOL			
	UNUSUAL ODOR			
	OTHER			
NEUROLOGICAL	IRRITABILITY			
	HYPERACTIVITY			
	INCREASED TANTRUMS			
	CLINGINESS			
	FAINTING			
	DIZZINESS			
	EXCESSIVE CRYING			
	LETHARGY/FATIGUE			
	MOTOR TICS			
	SEIZURES			
	DIFFICULTY SLEEPING			
	FEVER			
	LOW TEMPERATURE			
	OTHER			

DATE _____

MOM'S MEALS

BREAKFAST

SNACK

LUNCH

SNACK

DINNER

SNACK

MEDICATION

CHILD'S MEALS

BREAKFAST

SNACK

LUNCH

SNACK

DINNER

SNACK

MEDICATION

FOOD TRIALING: _____   DAYS TRIALED: _____

SYMPTOMS

	X	NOTES/TIME STARTED	NOTES

	Symptom	X	NOTES/TIME STARTED	NOTES
SKIN	ITCHINESS			
	HIVES			
	RASH			
	SWELLING			
	REDNESS			
	PALENESS			
	ECZEMA			
	OTHER			
THROAT STOMACH	DIFFICULTY SWALLOWING			
	CHOKING			
	REFLUX			
	IMMEDIATE VOMITING			
	DELAYED VOMITING			
	OTHER			
NASAL SINUSES	STUFFY NOSE			
	RUNNY NOSE			
	ITCHY THROAT			
	HOARSE VOICE			
	REPETITIVE COUGHING			
	OTHER			
LUNGS	WHEEZING			
	SHORTNESS OF BREATH			
	DIFFICULTY BREATHING			
	OTHER			
STOOL	DIARRHEA			
	CONSTIPATION			
	BLOODY STOOL			
	MUCOUS IN STOOL			
	GREEN STOOL			
	UNUSUAL ODOR			
	OTHER			
NEUROLOGICAL	IRRITABILITY			
	HYPERACTIVITY			
	INCREASED TANTRUMS			
	CLINGINESS			
	FAINTING			
	DIZZINESS			
	EXCESSIVE CRYING			
	LETHARGY/FATIGUE			
	MOTOR TICS			
	SEIZURES			
	DIFFICULTY SLEEPING			
	FEVER			
	LOW TEMPERATURE			
	OTHER			

DATE _____

MOM'S MEALS

BREAKFAST

SNACK

LUNCH

SNACK

DINNER

SNACK

MEDICATION

CHILD'S MEALS

BREAKFAST

SNACK

LUNCH

SNACK

DINNER

SNACK

MEDICATION

FOOD TRIALING: _____ DAYS TRIALED: _____

SYMPTOMS

		X	NOTES/TIME STARTED	NOTES

		X	NOTES/TIME STARTED	NOTES
SKIN	ITCHINESS			
	HIVES			
	RASH			
	SWELLING			
	REDNESS			
	PALENESS			
	ECZEMA			
	OTHER			
THROAT / STOMACH	DIFFICULTY SWALLOWING			
	CHOKING			
	REFLUX			
	IMMEDIATE VOMITING			
	DELAYED VOMITING			
	OTHER			
NASAL / SINUSES	STUFFY NOSE			
	RUNNY NOSE			
	ITCHY THROAT			
	HOARSE VOICE			
	REPETITIVE COUGHING			
	OTHER			
LUNGS	WHEEZING			
	SHORTNESS OF BREATH			
	DIFFICULTY BREATHING			
	OTHER			
STOOL	DIARRHEA			
	CONSTIPATION			
	BLOODY STOOL			
	MUCOUS IN STOOL			
	GREEN STOOL			
	UNUSUAL ODOR			
	OTHER			
NEUROLOGICAL	IRRITABILITY			
	HYPERACTIVITY			
	INCREASED TANTRUMS			
	CLINGINESS			
	FAINTING			
	DIZZINESS			
	EXCESSIVE CRYING			
	LETHARGY/FATIGUE			
	MOTOR TICS			
	SEIZURES			
	DIFFICULTY SLEEPING			
	FEVER			
	LOW TEMPERATURE			
	OTHER			

DATE _____

MOM'S MEALS
BREAKFAST

SNACK

LUNCH

SNACK

DINNER

SNACK

MEDICATION

CHILD'S MEALS
BREAKFAST

SNACK

LUNCH

SNACK

DINNER

SNACK

MEDICATION

FOOD TRIALING: _____ DAYS TRIALED: _____

SYMPTOMS

		X	NOTES/TIME STARTED	NOTES
SKIN	ITCHINESS			
	HIVES			
	RASH			
	SWELLING			
	REDNESS			
	PALENESS			
	ECZEMA			
	OTHER			
THROAT STOMACH	DIFFICULTY SWALLOWING			
	CHOKING			
	REFLUX			
	IMMEDIATE VOMITING			
	DELAYED VOMITING			
	OTHER			
NASAL SINUSES	STUFFY NOSE			
	RUNNY NOSE			
	ITCHY THROAT			
	HOARSE VOICE			
	REPETITIVE COUGHING			
	OTHER			
LUNGS	WHEEZING			
	SHORTNESS OF BREATH			
	DIFFICULTY BREATHING			
	OTHER			
STOOL	DIARRHEA			
	CONSTIPATION			
	BLOODY STOOL			
	MUCOUS IN STOOL			
	GREEN STOOL			
	UNUSUAL ODOR			
	OTHER			
NEUROLOGICAL	IRRITABILITY			
	HYPERACTIVITY			
	INCREASED TANTRUMS			
	CLINGINESS			
	FAINTING			
	DIZZINESS			
	EXCESSIVE CRYING			
	LETHARGY/FATIGUE			
	MOTOR TICS			
	SEIZURES			
	DIFFICULTY SLEEPING			
	FEVER			
	LOW TEMPERATURE			
	OTHER			

DATE _____

MOM'S MEALS
BREAKFAST

SNACK

LUNCH

SNACK

DINNER

SNACK

MEDICATION

CHILD'S MEALS
BREAKFAST

SNACK

LUNCH

SNACK

DINNER

SNACK

MEDICATION

FOOD TRIALING: _____   DAYS TRIALED: _____

SYMPTOMS

	Symptom	X	NOTES/TIME STARTED	NOTES
SKIN	ITCHINESS			
	HIVES			
	RASH			
	SWELLING			
	REDNESS			
	PALENESS			
	ECZEMA			
	OTHER			
THROAT STOMACH	DIFFICULTY SWALLOWING			
	CHOKING			
	REFLUX			
	IMMEDIATE VOMITING			
	DELAYED VOMITING			
	OTHER			
NASAL SINUSES	STUFFY NOSE			
	RUNNY NOSE			
	ITCHY THROAT			
	HOARSE VOICE			
	REPETITIVE COUGHING			
	OTHER			
LUNGS	WHEEZING			
	SHORTNESS OF BREATH			
	DIFFICULTY BREATHING			
	OTHER			
STOOL	DIARRHEA			
	CONSTIPATION			
	BLOODY STOOL			
	MUCOUS IN STOOL			
	GREEN STOOL			
	UNUSUAL ODOR			
	OTHER			
NEUROLOGICAL	IRRITABILITY			
	HYPERACTIVITY			
	INCREASED TANTRUMS			
	CLINGINESS			
	FAINTING			
	DIZZINESS			
	EXCESSIVE CRYING			
	LETHARGY/FATIGUE			
	MOTOR TICS			
	SEIZURES			
	DIFFICULTY SLEEPING			
	FEVER			
	LOW TEMPERATURE			
	OTHER			

DATE _____

MOM'S MEALS
BREAKFAST

SNACK
_____
_____
_____

LUNCH

SNACK
_____
_____
_____

DINNER

SNACK
_____
_____

MEDICATION
_____

CHILD'S MEALS
BREAKFAST

SNACK
_____
_____
_____

LUNCH

SNACK
_____
_____
_____

DINNER

SNACK
_____
_____

MEDICATION
_____

FOOD TRIALING: _____   DAYS TRIALED: _____

SYMPTOMS

		X	NOTES/TIME STARTED	NOTES

		X	NOTES/TIME STARTED	NOTES
SKIN	ITCHINESS			
	HIVES			
	RASH			
	SWELLING			
	REDNESS			
	PALENESS			
	ECZEMA			
	OTHER			
THROAT STOMACH	DIFFICULTY SWALLOWING			
	CHOKING			
	REFLUX			
	IMMEDIATE VOMITING			
	DELAYED VOMITING			
	OTHER			
NASAL SINUSES	STUFFY NOSE			
	RUNNY NOSE			
	ITCHY THROAT			
	HOARSE VOICE			
	REPETITIVE COUGHING			
	OTHER			
LUNGS	WHEEZING			
	SHORTNESS OF BREATH			
	DIFFICULTY BREATHING			
	OTHER			
STOOL	DIARRHEA			
	CONSTIPATION			
	BLOODY STOOL			
	MUCOUS IN STOOL			
	GREEN STOOL			
	UNUSUAL ODOR			
	OTHER			
NEUROLOGICAL	IRRITABILITY			
	HYPERACTIVITY			
	INCREASED TANTRUMS			
	CLINGINESS			
	FAINTING			
	DIZZINESS			
	EXCESSIVE CRYING			
	LETHARGY/FATIGUE			
	MOTOR TICS			
	SEIZURES			
	DIFFICULTY SLEEPING			
	FEVER			
	LOW TEMPERATURE			
	OTHER			

DATE _____

MOM'S MEALS
BREAKFAST

SNACK

LUNCH

SNACK

DINNER

SNACK

MEDICATION

CHILD'S MEALS
BREAKFAST

SNACK

LUNCH

SNACK

DINNER

SNACK

MEDICATION

FOOD TRIALING: _____ DAYS TRIALED: _____

SYMPTOMS

		X	NOTES/TIME STARTED	NOTES
SKIN	ITCHINESS			
	HIVES			
	RASH			
	SWELLING			
	REDNESS			
	PALENESS			
	ECZEMA			
	OTHER			
THROAT STOMACH	DIFFICULTY SWALLOWING			
	CHOKING			
	REFLUX			
	IMMEDIATE VOMITING			
	DELAYED VOMITING			
	OTHER			
NASAL SINUSES	STUFFY NOSE			
	RUNNY NOSE			
	ITCHY THROAT			
	HOARSE VOICE			
	REPETITIVE COUGHING			
	OTHER			
LUNGS	WHEEZING			
	SHORTNESS OF BREATH			
	DIFFICULTY BREATHING			
	OTHER			
STOOL	DIARRHEA			
	CONSTIPATION			
	BLOODY STOOL			
	MUCOUS IN STOOL			
	GREEN STOOL			
	UNUSUAL ODOR			
	OTHER			
NEUROLOGICAL	IRRITABILITY			
	HYPERACTIVITY			
	INCREASED TANTRUMS			
	CLINGINESS			
	FAINTING			
	DIZZINESS			
	EXCESSIVE CRYING			
	LETHARGY/FATIGUE			
	MOTOR TICS			
	SEIZURES			
	DIFFICULTY SLEEPING			
	FEVER			
	LOW TEMPERATURE			
	OTHER			

DATE _____

MOM'S MEALS

BREAKFAST

SNACK

LUNCH

SNACK

DINNER

SNACK

MEDICATION

CHILD'S MEALS

BREAKFAST

SNACK

LUNCH

SNACK

DINNER

SNACK

MEDICATION

FOOD TRIALING: _____ DAYS TRIALED: _____

SYMPTOMS

		X	NOTES/TIME STARTED	NOTES
SKIN	ITCHINESS			
	HIVES			
	RASH			
	SWELLING			
	REDNESS			
	PALENESS			
	ECZEMA			
	OTHER			
THROAT STOMACH	DIFFICULTY SWALLOWING			
	CHOKING			
	REFLUX			
	IMMEDIATE VOMITING			
	DELAYED VOMITING			
	OTHER			
NASAL SINUSES	STUFFY NOSE			
	RUNNY NOSE			
	ITCHY THROAT			
	HOARSE VOICE			
	REPETITIVE COUGHING			
	OTHER			
LUNGS	WHEEZING			
	SHORTNESS OF BREATH			
	DIFFICULTY BREATHING			
	OTHER			
STOOL	DIARRHEA			
	CONSTIPATION			
	BLOODY STOOL			
	MUCOUS IN STOOL			
	GREEN STOOL			
	UNUSUAL ODOR			
	OTHER			
NEUROLOGICAL	IRRITABILITY			
	HYPERACTIVITY			
	INCREASED TANTRUMS			
	CLINGINESS			
	FAINTING			
	DIZZINESS			
	EXCESSIVE CRYING			
	LETHARGY/FATIGUE			
	MOTOR TICS			
	SEIZURES			
	DIFFICULTY SLEEPING			
	FEVER			
	LOW TEMPERATURE			
	OTHER			

DATE _____

MOM'S MEALS

BREAKFAST

SNACK

LUNCH

SNACK

DINNER

SNACK

MEDICATION

CHILD'S MEALS

BREAKFAST

SNACK

LUNCH

SNACK

DINNER

SNACK

MEDICATION

FOOD TRIALING: _____ DAYS TRIALED: _____

SYMPTOMS

		X	NOTES/TIME STARTED	NOTES
SKIN	ITCHINESS			
	HIVES			
	RASH			
	SWELLING			
	REDNESS			
	PALENESS			
	ECZEMA			
	OTHER			
THROAT STOMACH	DIFFICULTY SWALLOWING			
	CHOKING			
	REFLUX			
	IMMEDIATE VOMITING			
	DELAYED VOMITING			
	OTHER			
NASAL SINUSES	STUFFY NOSE			
	RUNNY NOSE			
	ITCHY THROAT			
	HOARSE VOICE			
	REPETITIVE COUGHING			
	OTHER			
LUNGS	WHEEZING			
	SHORTNESS OF BREATH			
	DIFFICULTY BREATHING			
	OTHER			
STOOL	DIARRHEA			
	CONSTIPATION			
	BLOODY STOOL			
	MUCOUS IN STOOL			
	GREEN STOOL			
	UNUSUAL ODOR			
	OTHER			
NEUROLOGICAL	IRRITABILITY			
	HYPERACTIVITY			
	INCREASED TANTRUMS			
	CLINGINESS			
	FAINTING			
	DIZZINESS			
	EXCESSIVE CRYING			
	LETHARGY/FATIGUE			
	MOTOR TICS			
	SEIZURES			
	DIFFICULTY SLEEPING			
	FEVER			
	LOW TEMPERATURE			
	OTHER			

DATE _____

MOM'S MEALS

BREAKFAST

SNACK

LUNCH

SNACK

DINNER

SNACK

MEDICATION

CHILD'S MEALS

BREAKFAST

SNACK

LUNCH

SNACK

DINNER

SNACK

MEDICATION

FOOD TRIALING: _____ DAYS TRIALED: _____

SYMPTOMS

		X	NOTES/TIME STARTED	NOTES
SKIN	ITCHINESS			
	HIVES			
	RASH			
	SWELLING			
	REDNESS			
	PALENESS			
	ECZEMA			
	OTHER			
THROAT STOMACH	DIFFICULTY SWALLOWING			
	CHOKING			
	REFLUX			
	IMMEDIATE VOMITING			
	DELAYED VOMITING			
	OTHER			
NASAL SINUSES	STUFFY NOSE			
	RUNNY NOSE			
	ITCHY THROAT			
	HOARSE VOICE			
	REPETITIVE COUGHING			
	OTHER			
LUNGS	WHEEZING			
	SHORTNESS OF BREATH			
	DIFFICULTY BREATHING			
	OTHER			
STOOL	DIARRHEA			
	CONSTIPATION			
	BLOODY STOOL			
	MUCOUS IN STOOL			
	GREEN STOOL			
	UNUSUAL ODOR			
	OTHER			
NEUROLOGICAL	IRRITABILITY			
	HYPERACTIVITY			
	INCREASED TANTRUMS			
	CLINGINESS			
	FAINTING			
	DIZZINESS			
	EXCESSIVE CRYING			
	LETHARGY/FATIGUE			
	MOTOR TICS			
	SEIZURES			
	DIFFICULTY SLEEPING			
	FEVER			
	LOW TEMPERATURE			
	OTHER			

DATE _____

MOM'S MEALS

BREAKFAST

SNACK

LUNCH

SNACK

DINNER

SNACK

MEDICATION

CHILD'S MEALS

BREAKFAST

SNACK

LUNCH

SNACK

DINNER

SNACK

MEDICATION

FOOD TRIALING: _____ DAYS TRIALED: _____

SYMPTOMS

		X	NOTES/TIME STARTED	NOTES
SKIN	ITCHINESS			
	HIVES			
	RASH			
	SWELLING			
	REDNESS			
	PALENESS			
	ECZEMA			
	OTHER			
THROAT STOMACH	DIFFICULTY SWALLOWING			
	CHOKING			
	REFLUX			
	IMMEDIATE VOMITING			
	DELAYED VOMITING			
	OTHER			
NASAL SINUSES	STUFFY NOSE			
	RUNNY NOSE			
	ITCHY THROAT			
	HOARSE VOICE			
	REPETITIVE COUGHING			
	OTHER			
LUNGS	WHEEZING			
	SHORTNESS OF BREATH			
	DIFFICULTY BREATHING			
	OTHER			
STOOL	DIARRHEA			
	CONSTIPATION			
	BLOODY STOOL			
	MUCOUS IN STOOL			
	GREEN STOOL			
	UNUSUAL ODOR			
	OTHER			
NEUROLOGICAL	IRRITABILITY			
	HYPERACTIVITY			
	INCREASED TANTRUMS			
	CLINGINESS			
	FAINTING			
	DIZZINESS			
	EXCESSIVE CRYING			
	LETHARGY/FATIGUE			
	MOTOR TICS			
	SEIZURES			
	DIFFICULTY SLEEPING			
	FEVER			
	LOW TEMPERATURE			
	OTHER			

DATE _____

MOM'S MEALS

BREAKFAST

SNACK

LUNCH

SNACK

DINNER

SNACK

MEDICATION

CHILD'S MEALS

BREAKFAST

SNACK

LUNCH

SNACK

DINNER

SNACK

MEDICATION

FOOD TRIALING: _____ DAYS TRIALED: _____

SYMPTOMS

		X	NOTES/TIME STARTED	NOTES
SKIN	ITCHINESS			
	HIVES			
	RASH			
	SWELLING			
	REDNESS			
	PALENESS			
	ECZEMA			
	OTHER			
THROAT / STOMACH	DIFFICULTY SWALLOWING			
	CHOKING			
	REFLUX			
	IMMEDIATE VOMITING			
	DELAYED VOMITING			
	OTHER			
NASAL / SINUSES	STUFFY NOSE			
	RUNNY NOSE			
	ITCHY THROAT			
	HOARSE VOICE			
	REPETITIVE COUGHING			
	OTHER			
LUNGS	WHEEZING			
	SHORTNESS OF BREATH			
	DIFFICULTY BREATHING			
	OTHER			
STOOL	DIARRHEA			
	CONSTIPATION			
	BLOODY STOOL			
	MUCOUS IN STOOL			
	GREEN STOOL			
	UNUSUAL ODOR			
	OTHER			
NEUROLOGICAL	IRRITABILITY			
	HYPERACTIVITY			
	INCREASED TANTRUMS			
	CLINGINESS			
	FAINTING			
	DIZZINESS			
	EXCESSIVE CRYING			
	LETHARGY/FATIGUE			
	MOTOR TICS			
	SEIZURES			
	DIFFICULTY SLEEPING			
	FEVER			
	LOW TEMPERATURE			
	OTHER			

DATE _____

MOM'S MEALS
BREAKFAST

SNACK

LUNCH

SNACK

DINNER

SNACK

MEDICATION

CHILD'S MEALS
BREAKFAST

SNACK

LUNCH

SNACK

DINNER

SNACK

MEDICATION

FOOD TRIALING: _____   DAYS TRIALED: _____

SYMPTOMS

		X	NOTES/TIME STARTED	NOTES
SKIN	ITCHINESS			
	HIVES			
	RASH			
	SWELLING			
	REDNESS			
	PALENESS			
	ECZEMA			
	OTHER			
THROAT STOMACH	DIFFICULTY SWALLOWING			
	CHOKING			
	REFLUX			
	IMMEDIATE VOMITING			
	DELAYED VOMITING			
	OTHER			
NASAL SINUSES	STUFFY NOSE			
	RUNNY NOSE			
	ITCHY THROAT			
	HOARSE VOICE			
	REPETITIVE COUGHING			
	OTHER			
LUNGS	WHEEZING			
	SHORTNESS OF BREATH			
	DIFFICULTY BREATHING			
	OTHER			
STOOL	DIARRHEA			
	CONSTIPATION			
	BLOODY STOOL			
	MUCOUS IN STOOL			
	GREEN STOOL			
	UNUSUAL ODOR			
	OTHER			
NEUROLOGICAL	IRRITABILITY			
	HYPERACTIVITY			
	INCREASED TANTRUMS			
	CLINGINESS			
	FAINTING			
	DIZZINESS			
	EXCESSIVE CRYING			
	LETHARGY/FATIGUE			
	MOTOR TICS			
	SEIZURES			
	DIFFICULTY SLEEPING			
	FEVER			
	LOW TEMPERATURE			
	OTHER			

DATE _____

MOM'S MEALS

BREAKFAST

SNACK

LUNCH

SNACK

DINNER

SNACK

MEDICATION

CHILD'S MEALS

BREAKFAST

SNACK

LUNCH

SNACK

DINNER

SNACK

MEDICATION

FOOD TRIALING: _____ DAYS TRIALED: _____

SYMPTOMS

	SYMPTOM	X	NOTES/TIME STARTED	NOTES
SKIN	ITCHINESS			
	HIVES			
	RASH			
	SWELLING			
	REDNESS			
	PALENESS			
	ECZEMA			
	OTHER			
THROAT STOMACH	DIFFICULTY SWALLOWING			
	CHOKING			
	REFLUX			
	IMMEDIATE VOMITING			
	DELAYED VOMITING			
	OTHER			
NASAL SINUSES	STUFFY NOSE			
	RUNNY NOSE			
	ITCHY THROAT			
	HOARSE VOICE			
	REPETITIVE COUGHING			
	OTHER			
LUNGS	WHEEZING			
	SHORTNESS OF BREATH			
	DIFFICULTY BREATHING			
	OTHER			
STOOL	DIARRHEA			
	CONSTIPATION			
	BLOODY STOOL			
	MUCOUS IN STOOL			
	GREEN STOOL			
	UNUSUAL ODOR			
	OTHER			
NEUROLOGICAL	IRRITABILITY			
	HYPERACTIVITY			
	INCREASED TANTRUMS			
	CLINGINESS			
	FAINTING			
	DIZZINESS			
	EXCESSIVE CRYING			
	LETHARGY/FATIGUE			
	MOTOR TICS			
	SEIZURES			
	DIFFICULTY SLEEPING			
	FEVER			
	LOW TEMPERATURE			
	OTHER			

DATE _____

MOM'S MEALS
BREAKFAST

SNACK

LUNCH

SNACK

DINNER

SNACK

MEDICATION

CHILD'S MEALS
BREAKFAST

SNACK

LUNCH

SNACK

DINNER

SNACK

MEDICATION

FOOD TRIALING: _____ DAYS TRIALED: _____

SYMPTOMS

	Symptom	X	NOTES/TIME STARTED	NOTES
SKIN	ITCHINESS			
	HIVES			
	RASH			
	SWELLING			
	REDNESS			
	PALENESS			
	ECZEMA			
	OTHER			
THROAT STOMACH	DIFFICULTY SWALLOWING			
	CHOKING			
	REFLUX			
	IMMEDIATE VOMITING			
	DELAYED VOMITING			
	OTHER			
NASAL SINUSES	STUFFY NOSE			
	RUNNY NOSE			
	ITCHY THROAT			
	HOARSE VOICE			
	REPETITIVE COUGHING			
	OTHER			
LUNGS	WHEEZING			
	SHORTNESS OF BREATH			
	DIFFICULTY BREATHING			
	OTHER			
STOOL	DIARRHEA			
	CONSTIPATION			
	BLOODY STOOL			
	MUCOUS IN STOOL			
	GREEN STOOL			
	UNUSUAL ODOR			
	OTHER			
NEUROLOGICAL	IRRITABILITY			
	HYPERACTIVITY			
	INCREASED TANTRUMS			
	CLINGINESS			
	FAINTING			
	DIZZINESS			
	EXCESSIVE CRYING			
	LETHARGY/FATIGUE			
	MOTOR TICS			
	SEIZURES			
	DIFFICULTY SLEEPING			
	FEVER			
	LOW TEMPERATURE			
	OTHER			

DATE _____

MOM'S MEALS

BREAKFAST

SNACK

LUNCH

SNACK

DINNER

SNACK

MEDICATION

CHILD'S MEALS

BREAKFAST

SNACK

LUNCH

SNACK

DINNER

SNACK

MEDICATION

FOOD TRIALING: _____ DAYS TRIALED: _____

SYMPTOMS

		X	NOTES/TIME STARTED	NOTES
SKIN	ITCHINESS			
	HIVES			
	RASH			
	SWELLING			
	REDNESS			
	PALENESS			
	ECZEMA			
	OTHER			
THROAT STOMACH	DIFFICULTY SWALLOWING			
	CHOKING			
	REFLUX			
	IMMEDIATE VOMITING			
	DELAYED VOMITING			
	OTHER			
NASAL SINUSES	STUFFY NOSE			
	RUNNY NOSE			
	ITCHY THROAT			
	HOARSE VOICE			
	REPETITIVE COUGHING			
	OTHER			
LUNGS	WHEEZING			
	SHORTNESS OF BREATH			
	DIFFICULTY BREATHING			
	OTHER			
STOOL	DIARRHEA			
	CONSTIPATION			
	BLOODY STOOL			
	MUCOUS IN STOOL			
	GREEN STOOL			
	UNUSUAL ODOR			
	OTHER			
NEUROLOGICAL	IRRITABILITY			
	HYPERACTIVITY			
	INCREASED TANTRUMS			
	CLINGINESS			
	FAINTING			
	DIZZINESS			
	EXCESSIVE CRYING			
	LETHARGY/FATIGUE			
	MOTOR TICS			
	SEIZURES			
	DIFFICULTY SLEEPING			
	FEVER			
	LOW TEMPERATURE			
	OTHER			

DATE _____

MOM'S MEALS
BREAKFAST

SNACK
_____
_____
_____

LUNCH

SNACK
_____
_____
_____

DINNER

SNACK
_____
_____
_____

MEDICATION

CHILD'S MEALS
BREAKFAST

SNACK
_____
_____
_____

LUNCH

SNACK
_____
_____
_____

DINNER

SNACK
_____
_____
_____

MEDICATION

FOOD TRIALING: _____ DAYS TRIALED: _____

SYMPTOMS

		X	NOTES/TIME STARTED	NOTES
SKIN	ITCHINESS			
	HIVES			
	RASH			
	SWELLING			
	REDNESS			
	PALENESS			
	ECZEMA			
	OTHER			
THROAT STOMACH	DIFFICULTY SWALLOWING			
	CHOKING			
	REFLUX			
	IMMEDIATE VOMITING			
	DELAYED VOMITING			
	OTHER			
NASAL SINUSES	STUFFY NOSE			
	RUNNY NOSE			
	ITCHY THROAT			
	HOARSE VOICE			
	REPETITIVE COUGHING			
	OTHER			
LUNGS	WHEEZING			
	SHORTNESS OF BREATH			
	DIFFICULTY BREATHING			
	OTHER			
STOOL	DIARRHEA			
	CONSTIPATION			
	BLOODY STOOL			
	MUCOUS IN STOOL			
	GREEN STOOL			
	UNUSUAL ODOR			
	OTHER			
NEUROLOGICAL	IRRITABILITY			
	HYPERACTIVITY			
	INCREASED TANTRUMS			
	CLINGINESS			
	FAINTING			
	DIZZINESS			
	EXCESSIVE CRYING			
	LETHARGY/FATIGUE			
	MOTOR TICS			
	SEIZURES			
	DIFFICULTY SLEEPING			
	FEVER			
	LOW TEMPERATURE			
	OTHER			

DATE _____

MOM'S MEALS

BREAKFAST

SNACK

LUNCH

SNACK

DINNER

SNACK

MEDICATION

CHILD'S MEALS

BREAKFAST

SNACK

LUNCH

SNACK

DINNER

SNACK

MEDICATION

FOOD TRIALING: _____ DAYS TRIALED: _____

SYMPTOMS

		X	NOTES/TIME STARTED	NOTES
SKIN	ITCHINESS			
	HIVES			
	RASH			
	SWELLING			
	REDNESS			
	PALENESS			
	ECZEMA			
	OTHER			
THROAT STOMACH	DIFFICULTY SWALLOWING			
	CHOKING			
	REFLUX			
	IMMEDIATE VOMITING			
	DELAYED VOMITING			
	OTHER			
NASAL SINUSES	STUFFY NOSE			
	RUNNY NOSE			
	ITCHY THROAT			
	HOARSE VOICE			
	REPETITIVE COUGHING			
	OTHER			
LUNGS	WHEEZING			
	SHORTNESS OF BREATH			
	DIFFICULTY BREATHING			
	OTHER			
STOOL	DIARRHEA			
	CONSTIPATION			
	BLOODY STOOL			
	MUCOUS IN STOOL			
	GREEN STOOL			
	UNUSUAL ODOR			
	OTHER			
NEUROLOGICAL	IRRITABILITY			
	HYPERACTIVITY			
	INCREASED TANTRUMS			
	CLINGINESS			
	FAINTING			
	DIZZINESS			
	EXCESSIVE CRYING			
	LETHARGY/FATIGUE			
	MOTOR TICS			
	SEIZURES			
	DIFFICULTY SLEEPING			
	FEVER			
	LOW TEMPERATURE			
	OTHER			

DATE _____

MOM'S MEALS

BREAKFAST

SNACK

LUNCH

SNACK

DINNER

SNACK

MEDICATION

CHILD'S MEALS

BREAKFAST

SNACK

LUNCH

SNACK

DINNER

SNACK

MEDICATION

FOOD TRIALING: _____ DAYS TRIALED: _____

SYMPTOMS

		X	NOTES/TIME STARTED	NOTES
SKIN	ITCHINESS			
	HIVES			
	RASH			
	SWELLING			
	REDNESS			
	PALENESS			
	ECZEMA			
	OTHER			
THROAT STOMACH	DIFFICULTY SWALLOWING			
	CHOKING			
	REFLUX			
	IMMEDIATE VOMITING			
	DELAYED VOMITING			
	OTHER			
NASAL SINUSES	STUFFY NOSE			
	RUNNY NOSE			
	ITCHY THROAT			
	HOARSE VOICE			
	REPETITIVE COUGHING			
	OTHER			
LUNGS	WHEEZING			
	SHORTNESS OF BREATH			
	DIFFICULTY BREATHING			
	OTHER			
STOOL	DIARRHEA			
	CONSTIPATION			
	BLOODY STOOL			
	MUCOUS IN STOOL			
	GREEN STOOL			
	UNUSUAL ODOR			
	OTHER			
NEUROLOGICAL	IRRITABILITY			
	HYPERACTIVITY			
	INCREASED TANTRUMS			
	CLINGINESS			
	FAINTING			
	DIZZINESS			
	EXCESSIVE CRYING			
	LETHARGY/FATIGUE			
	MOTOR TICS			
	SEIZURES			
	DIFFICULTY SLEEPING			
	FEVER			
	LOW TEMPERATURE			
	OTHER			

DATE _____

MOM'S MEALS

BREAKFAST

SNACK

LUNCH

SNACK

DINNER

SNACK

MEDICATION

CHILD'S MEALS

BREAKFAST

SNACK

LUNCH

SNACK

DINNER

SNACK

MEDICATION

FOOD TRIALING: _____ DAYS TRIALED: _____

SYMPTOMS

	SYMPTOMS	X	NOTES/TIME STARTED	NOTES
SKIN	ITCHINESS			
	HIVES			
	RASH			
	SWELLING			
	REDNESS			
	PALENESS			
	ECZEMA			
	OTHER			
THROAT STOMACH	DIFFICULTY SWALLOWING			
	CHOKING			
	REFLUX			
	IMMEDIATE VOMITING			
	DELAYED VOMITING			
	OTHER			
NASAL SINUSES	STUFFY NOSE			
	RUNNY NOSE			
	ITCHY THROAT			
	HOARSE VOICE			
	REPETITIVE COUGHING			
	OTHER			
LUNGS	WHEEZING			
	SHORTNESS OF BREATH			
	DIFFICULTY BREATHING			
	OTHER			
STOOL	DIARRHEA			
	CONSTIPATION			
	BLOODY STOOL			
	MUCOUS IN STOOL			
	GREEN STOOL			
	UNUSUAL ODOR			
	OTHER			
NEUROLOGICAL	IRRITABILITY			
	HYPERACTIVITY			
	INCREASED TANTRUMS			
	CLINGINESS			
	FAINTING			
	DIZZINESS			
	EXCESSIVE CRYING			
	LETHARGY/FATIGUE			
	MOTOR TICS			
	SEIZURES			
	DIFFICULTY SLEEPING			
	FEVER			
	LOW TEMPERATURE			
	OTHER			

DATE _____

MOM'S MEALS

BREAKFAST

SNACK

LUNCH

SNACK

DINNER

SNACK

MEDICATION

CHILD'S MEALS

BREAKFAST

SNACK

LUNCH

SNACK

DINNER

SNACK

MEDICATION

FOOD TRIALING: _____ DAYS TRIALED: _____

SYMPTOMS

	Symptom	X	NOTES/TIME STARTED	NOTES
SKIN	ITCHINESS			
	HIVES			
	RASH			
	SWELLING			
	REDNESS			
	PALENESS			
	ECZEMA			
	OTHER			
THROAT STOMACH	DIFFICULTY SWALLOWING			
	CHOKING			
	REFLUX			
	IMMEDIATE VOMITING			
	DELAYED VOMITING			
	OTHER			
NASAL SINUSES	STUFFY NOSE			
	RUNNY NOSE			
	ITCHY THROAT			
	HOARSE VOICE			
	REPETITIVE COUGHING			
	OTHER			
LUNGS	WHEEZING			
	SHORTNESS OF BREATH			
	DIFFICULTY BREATHING			
	OTHER			
STOOL	DIARRHEA			
	CONSTIPATION			
	BLOODY STOOL			
	MUCOUS IN STOOL			
	GREEN STOOL			
	UNUSUAL ODOR			
	OTHER			
NEUROLOGICAL	IRRITABILITY			
	HYPERACTIVITY			
	INCREASED TANTRUMS			
	CLINGINESS			
	FAINTING			
	DIZZINESS			
	EXCESSIVE CRYING			
	LETHARGY/FATIGUE			
	MOTOR TICS			
	SEIZURES			
	DIFFICULTY SLEEPING			
	FEVER			
	LOW TEMPERATURE			
	OTHER			

DATE _____

MOM'S MEALS

BREAKFAST

SNACK _____

LUNCH

SNACK _____

DINNER

SNACK _____

MEDICATION

CHILD'S MEALS

BREAKFAST

SNACK _____

LUNCH

SNACK _____

DINNER

SNACK _____

MEDICATION

FOOD TRIALING: _____ DAYS TRIALED: _____

SYMPTOMS

		X	NOTES/TIME STARTED	NOTES
SKIN	ITCHINESS			
	HIVES			
	RASH			
	SWELLING			
	REDNESS			
	PALENESS			
	ECZEMA			
	OTHER			
THROAT / STOMACH	DIFFICULTY SWALLOWING			
	CHOKING			
	REFLUX			
	IMMEDIATE VOMITING			
	DELAYED VOMITING			
	OTHER			
NASAL / SINUSES	STUFFY NOSE			
	RUNNY NOSE			
	ITCHY THROAT			
	HOARSE VOICE			
	REPETITIVE COUGHING			
	OTHER			
LUNGS	WHEEZING			
	SHORTNESS OF BREATH			
	DIFFICULTY BREATHING			
	OTHER			
STOOL	DIARRHEA			
	CONSTIPATION			
	BLOODY STOOL			
	MUCOUS IN STOOL			
	GREEN STOOL			
	UNUSUAL ODOR			
	OTHER			
NEUROLOGICAL	IRRITABILITY			
	HYPERACTIVITY			
	INCREASED TANTRUMS			
	CLINGINESS			
	FAINTING			
	DIZZINESS			
	EXCESSIVE CRYING			
	LETHARGY/FATIGUE			
	MOTOR TICS			
	SEIZURES			
	DIFFICULTY SLEEPING			
	FEVER			
	LOW TEMPERATURE			
	OTHER			

DATE _____

MOM'S MEALS
BREAKFAST

SNACK
_____

LUNCH

SNACK
_____

DINNER

SNACK
_____

MEDICATION

CHILD'S MEALS
BREAKFAST

SNACK
_____

LUNCH

SNACK
_____

DINNER

SNACK
_____

MEDICATION

FOOD TRIALING: _____   DAYS TRIALED: _____

SYMPTOMS

	Symptom	X	NOTES/TIME STARTED	NOTES
SKIN	ITCHINESS			
	HIVES			
	RASH			
	SWELLING			
	REDNESS			
	PALENESS			
	ECZEMA			
	OTHER			
THROAT / STOMACH	DIFFICULTY SWALLOWING			
	CHOKING			
	REFLUX			
	IMMEDIATE VOMITING			
	DELAYED VOMITING			
	OTHER			
NASAL / SINUSES	STUFFY NOSE			
	RUNNY NOSE			
	ITCHY THROAT			
	HOARSE VOICE			
	REPETITIVE COUGHING			
	OTHER			
LUNGS	WHEEZING			
	SHORTNESS OF BREATH			
	DIFFICULTY BREATHING			
	OTHER			
STOOL	DIARRHEA			
	CONSTIPATION			
	BLOODY STOOL			
	MUCOUS IN STOOL			
	GREEN STOOL			
	UNUSUAL ODOR			
	OTHER			
NEUROLOGICAL	IRRITABILITY			
	HYPERACTIVITY			
	INCREASED TANTRUMS			
	CLINGINESS			
	FAINTING			
	DIZZINESS			
	EXCESSIVE CRYING			
	LETHARGY/FATIGUE			
	MOTOR TICS			
	SEIZURES			
	DIFFICULTY SLEEPING			
	FEVER			
	LOW TEMPERATURE			
	OTHER			

DATE _____

MOM'S MEALS
BREAKFAST

SNACK

LUNCH

SNACK

DINNER

SNACK

MEDICATION

CHILD'S MEALS
BREAKFAST

SNACK

LUNCH

SNACK

DINNER

SNACK

MEDICATION

FOOD TRIALING: _____ DAYS TRIALED: _____

SYMPTOMS

		X	NOTES/TIME STARTED	NOTES
SKIN	ITCHINESS			
	HIVES			
	RASH			
	SWELLING			
	REDNESS			
	PALENESS			
	ECZEMA			
	OTHER			
THROAT STOMACH	DIFFICULTY SWALLOWING			
	CHOKING			
	REFLUX			
	IMMEDIATE VOMITING			
	DELAYED VOMITING			
	OTHER			
NASAL SINUSES	STUFFY NOSE			
	RUNNY NOSE			
	ITCHY THROAT			
	HOARSE VOICE			
	REPETITIVE COUGHING			
	OTHER			
LUNGS	WHEEZING			
	SHORTNESS OF BREATH			
	DIFFICULTY BREATHING			
	OTHER			
STOOL	DIARRHEA			
	CONSTIPATION			
	BLOODY STOOL			
	MUCOUS IN STOOL			
	GREEN STOOL			
	UNUSUAL ODOR			
	OTHER			
NEUROLOGICAL	IRRITABILITY			
	HYPERACTIVITY			
	INCREASED TANTRUMS			
	CLINGINESS			
	FAINTING			
	DIZZINESS			
	EXCESSIVE CRYING			
	LETHARGY/FATIGUE			
	MOTOR TICS			
	SEIZURES			
	DIFFICULTY SLEEPING			
	FEVER			
	LOW TEMPERATURE			
	OTHER			

DATE _____

MOM'S MEALS

CHILD'S MEALS

BREAKFAST

BREAKFAST

SNACK _____

SNACK _____

LUNCH

LUNCH

SNACK _____

SNACK _____

DINNER

DINNER

SNACK _____

SNACK _____

MEDICATION

MEDICATION

FOOD TRIALING: _____   DAYS TRIALED: _____

SYMPTOMS

		X	NOTES/TIME STARTED	NOTES

		X NOTES/TIME STARTED	NOTES
SKIN	ITCHINESS		
	HIVES		
	RASH		
	SWELLING		
	REDNESS		
	PALENESS		
	ECZEMA		
	OTHER		
THROAT STOMACH	DIFFICULTY SWALLOWING		
	CHOKING		
	REFLUX		
	IMMEDIATE VOMITING		
	DELAYED VOMITING		
	OTHER		
NASAL SINUSES	STUFFY NOSE		
	RUNNY NOSE		
	ITCHY THROAT		
	HOARSE VOICE		
	REPETITIVE COUGHING		
	OTHER		
LUNGS	WHEEZING		
	SHORTNESS OF BREATH		
	DIFFICULTY BREATHING		
	OTHER		
STOOL	DIARRHEA		
	CONSTIPATION		
	BLOODY STOOL		
	MUCOUS IN STOOL		
	GREEN STOOL		
	UNUSUAL ODOR		
	OTHER		
NEUROLOGICAL	IRRITABILITY		
	HYPERACTIVITY		
	INCREASED TANTRUMS		
	CLINGINESS		
	FAINTING		
	DIZZINESS		
	EXCESSIVE CRYING		
	LETHARGY/FATIGUE		
	MOTOR TICS		
	SEIZURES		
	DIFFICULTY SLEEPING		
	FEVER		
	LOW TEMPERATURE		
	OTHER		

DATE _____

MOM'S MEALS
BREAKFAST

SNACK

LUNCH

SNACK

DINNER

SNACK

MEDICATION

CHILD'S MEALS
BREAKFAST

SNACK

LUNCH

SNACK

DINNER

SNACK

MEDICATION

FOOD TRIALING: _____   DAYS TRIALED: _____

SYMPTOMS

	Symptom	X	NOTES/TIME STARTED	NOTES
SKIN	ITCHINESS			
	HIVES			
	RASH			
	SWELLING			
	REDNESS			
	PALENESS			
	ECZEMA			
	OTHER			
THROAT STOMACH	DIFFICULTY SWALLOWING			
	CHOKING			
	REFLUX			
	IMMEDIATE VOMITING			
	DELAYED VOMITING			
	OTHER			
NASAL SINUSES	STUFFY NOSE			
	RUNNY NOSE			
	ITCHY THROAT			
	HOARSE VOICE			
	REPETITIVE COUGHING			
	OTHER			
LUNGS	WHEEZING			
	SHORTNESS OF BREATH			
	DIFFICULTY BREATHING			
	OTHER			
STOOL	DIARRHEA			
	CONSTIPATION			
	BLOODY STOOL			
	MUCOUS IN STOOL			
	GREEN STOOL			
	UNUSUAL ODOR			
	OTHER			
NEUROLOGICAL	IRRITABILITY			
	HYPERACTIVITY			
	INCREASED TANTRUMS			
	CLINGINESS			
	FAINTING			
	DIZZINESS			
	EXCESSIVE CRYING			
	LETHARGY/FATIGUE			
	MOTOR TICS			
	SEIZURES			
	DIFFICULTY SLEEPING			
	FEVER			
	LOW TEMPERATURE			
	OTHER			

DATE _____

MOM'S MEALS

BREAKFAST

SNACK

LUNCH

SNACK

DINNER

SNACK

MEDICATION

CHILD'S MEALS

BREAKFAST

SNACK

LUNCH

SNACK

DINNER

SNACK

MEDICATION

FOOD TRIALING: _____   DAYS TRIALED: _____

SYMPTOMS

	Symptom	X	NOTES/TIME STARTED	NOTES
SKIN	ITCHINESS			
	HIVES			
	RASH			
	SWELLING			
	REDNESS			
	PALENESS			
	ECZEMA			
	OTHER			
THROAT / STOMACH	DIFFICULTY SWALLOWING			
	CHOKING			
	REFLUX			
	IMMEDIATE VOMITING			
	DELAYED VOMITING			
	OTHER			
NASAL / SINUSES	STUFFY NOSE			
	RUNNY NOSE			
	ITCHY THROAT			
	HOARSE VOICE			
	REPETITIVE COUGHING			
	OTHER			
LUNGS	WHEEZING			
	SHORTNESS OF BREATH			
	DIFFICULTY BREATHING			
	OTHER			
STOOL	DIARRHEA			
	CONSTIPATION			
	BLOODY STOOL			
	MUCOUS IN STOOL			
	GREEN STOOL			
	UNUSUAL ODOR			
	OTHER			
NEUROLOGICAL	IRRITABILITY			
	HYPERACTIVITY			
	INCREASED TANTRUMS			
	CLINGINESS			
	FAINTING			
	DIZZINESS			
	EXCESSIVE CRYING			
	LETHARGY/FATIGUE			
	MOTOR TICS			
	SEIZURES			
	DIFFICULTY SLEEPING			
	FEVER			
	LOW TEMPERATURE			
	OTHER			

DATE _____

MOM'S MEALS
BREAKFAST

SNACK

LUNCH

SNACK

DINNER

SNACK

MEDICATION

CHILD'S MEALS
BREAKFAST

SNACK

LUNCH

SNACK

DINNER

SNACK

MEDICATION

FOOD TRIALING: _____ DAYS TRIALED: _____

SYMPTOMS

		X	NOTES/TIME STARTED	NOTES
SKIN	ITCHINESS			
	HIVES			
	RASH			
	SWELLING			
	REDNESS			
	PALENESS			
	ECZEMA			
	OTHER			
THROAT STOMACH	DIFFICULTY SWALLOWING			
	CHOKING			
	REFLUX			
	IMMEDIATE VOMITING			
	DELAYED VOMITING			
	OTHER			
NASAL SINUSES	STUFFY NOSE			
	RUNNY NOSE			
	ITCHY THROAT			
	HOARSE VOICE			
	REPETITIVE COUGHING			
	OTHER			
LUNGS	WHEEZING			
	SHORTNESS OF BREATH			
	DIFFICULTY BREATHING			
	OTHER			
STOOL	DIARRHEA			
	CONSTIPATION			
	BLOODY STOOL			
	MUCOUS IN STOOL			
	GREEN STOOL			
	UNUSUAL ODOR			
	OTHER			
NEUROLOGICAL	IRRITABILITY			
	HYPERACTIVITY			
	INCREASED TANTRUMS			
	CLINGINESS			
	FAINTING			
	DIZZINESS			
	EXCESSIVE CRYING			
	LETHARGY/FATIGUE			
	MOTOR TICS			
	SEIZURES			
	DIFFICULTY SLEEPING			
	FEVER			
	LOW TEMPERATURE			
	OTHER			

DATE _____

MOM'S MEALS

BREAKFAST

SNACK

LUNCH

SNACK

DINNER

SNACK

MEDICATION

CHILD'S MEALS

BREAKFAST

SNACK

LUNCH

SNACK

DINNER

SNACK

MEDICATION

FOOD TRIALING: _____ DAYS TRIALED: _____

SYMPTOMS

		X	NOTES/TIME STARTED	NOTES

		X	NOTES/TIME STARTED	NOTES
SKIN	ITCHINESS			
	HIVES			
	RASH			
	SWELLING			
	REDNESS			
	PALENESS			
	ECZEMA			
	OTHER			
THROAT STOMACH	DIFFICULTY SWALLOWING			
	CHOKING			
	REFLUX			
	IMMEDIATE VOMITING			
	DELAYED VOMITING			
	OTHER			
NASAL SINUSES	STUFFY NOSE			
	RUNNY NOSE			
	ITCHY THROAT			
	HOARSE VOICE			
	REPETITIVE COUGHING			
	OTHER			
LUNGS	WHEEZING			
	SHORTNESS OF BREATH			
	DIFFICULTY BREATHING			
	OTHER			
STOOL	DIARRHEA			
	CONSTIPATION			
	BLOODY STOOL			
	MUCOUS IN STOOL			
	GREEN STOOL			
	UNUSUAL ODOR			
	OTHER			
NEUROLOGICAL	IRRITABILITY			
	HYPERACTIVITY			
	INCREASED TANTRUMS			
	CLINGINESS			
	FAINTING			
	DIZZINESS			
	EXCESSIVE CRYING			
	LETHARGY/FATIGUE			
	MOTOR TICS			
	SEIZURES			
	DIFFICULTY SLEEPING			
	FEVER			
	LOW TEMPERATURE			
	OTHER			

DATE _____

MOM'S MEALS

BREAKFAST

SNACK

LUNCH

SNACK

DINNER

SNACK

MEDICATION

CHILD'S MEALS

BREAKFAST

SNACK

LUNCH

SNACK

DINNER

SNACK

MEDICATION

FOOD TRIALING: _____ DAYS TRIALED: _____

SYMPTOMS

		X	NOTES/TIME STARTED	NOTES
SKIN	ITCHINESS			
	HIVES			
	RASH			
	SWELLING			
	REDNESS			
	PALENESS			
	ECZEMA			
	OTHER			
THROAT / STOMACH	DIFFICULTY SWALLOWING			
	CHOKING			
	REFLUX			
	IMMEDIATE VOMITING			
	DELAYED VOMITING			
	OTHER			
NASAL / SINUSES	STUFFY NOSE			
	RUNNY NOSE			
	ITCHY THROAT			
	HOARSE VOICE			
	REPETITIVE COUGHING			
	OTHER			
LUNGS	WHEEZING			
	SHORTNESS OF BREATH			
	DIFFICULTY BREATHING			
	OTHER			
STOOL	DIARRHEA			
	CONSTIPATION			
	BLOODY STOOL			
	MUCOUS IN STOOL			
	GREEN STOOL			
	UNUSUAL ODOR			
	OTHER			
NEUROLOGICAL	IRRITABILITY			
	HYPERACTIVITY			
	INCREASED TANTRUMS			
	CLINGINESS			
	FAINTING			
	DIZZINESS			
	EXCESSIVE CRYING			
	LETHARGY/FATIGUE			
	MOTOR TICS			
	SEIZURES			
	DIFFICULTY SLEEPING			
	FEVER			
	LOW TEMPERATURE			
	OTHER			

DATE _____

MOM'S MEALS

BREAKFAST

SNACK

LUNCH

SNACK

DINNER

SNACK

MEDICATION

CHILD'S MEALS

BREAKFAST

SNACK

LUNCH

SNACK

DINNER

SNACK

MEDICATION

FOOD TRIALING: _____   DAYS TRIALED: _____

SYMPTOMS

		X	NOTES/TIME STARTED	NOTES
SKIN	ITCHINESS			
	HIVES			
	RASH			
	SWELLING			
	REDNESS			
	PALENESS			
	ECZEMA			
	OTHER			
THROAT STOMACH	DIFFICULTY SWALLOWING			
	CHOKING			
	REFLUX			
	IMMEDIATE VOMITING			
	DELAYED VOMITING			
	OTHER			
NASAL SINUSES	STUFFY NOSE			
	RUNNY NOSE			
	ITCHY THROAT			
	HOARSE VOICE			
	REPETITIVE COUGHING			
	OTHER			
LUNGS	WHEEZING			
	SHORTNESS OF BREATH			
	DIFFICULTY BREATHING			
	OTHER			
STOOL	DIARRHEA			
	CONSTIPATION			
	BLOODY STOOL			
	MUCOUS IN STOOL			
	GREEN STOOL			
	UNUSUAL ODOR			
	OTHER			
NEUROLOGICAL	IRRITABILITY			
	HYPERACTIVITY			
	INCREASED TANTRUMS			
	CLINGINESS			
	FAINTING			
	DIZZINESS			
	EXCESSIVE CRYING			
	LETHARGY/FATIGUE			
	MOTOR TICS			
	SEIZURES			
	DIFFICULTY SLEEPING			
	FEVER			
	LOW TEMPERATURE			
	OTHER			

NOTES/CONCERNS TO DISCUSS WITH THE DOCTOR

DATE OF NEXT APPOINTMENT: _____

TOPICS/CONCERNS TO DISCUSS:

NOTES

NOTES

NOTES

Made in the USA
Coppell, TX
07 October 2020